MONROE COLLEGE LIBRARY
3 7340 00004993 9

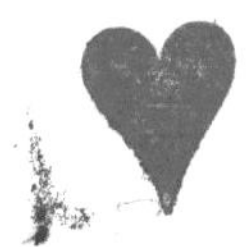

LIBRARY
MONROE COLLEGE
NEW ROCHELLE, NY

D1528430

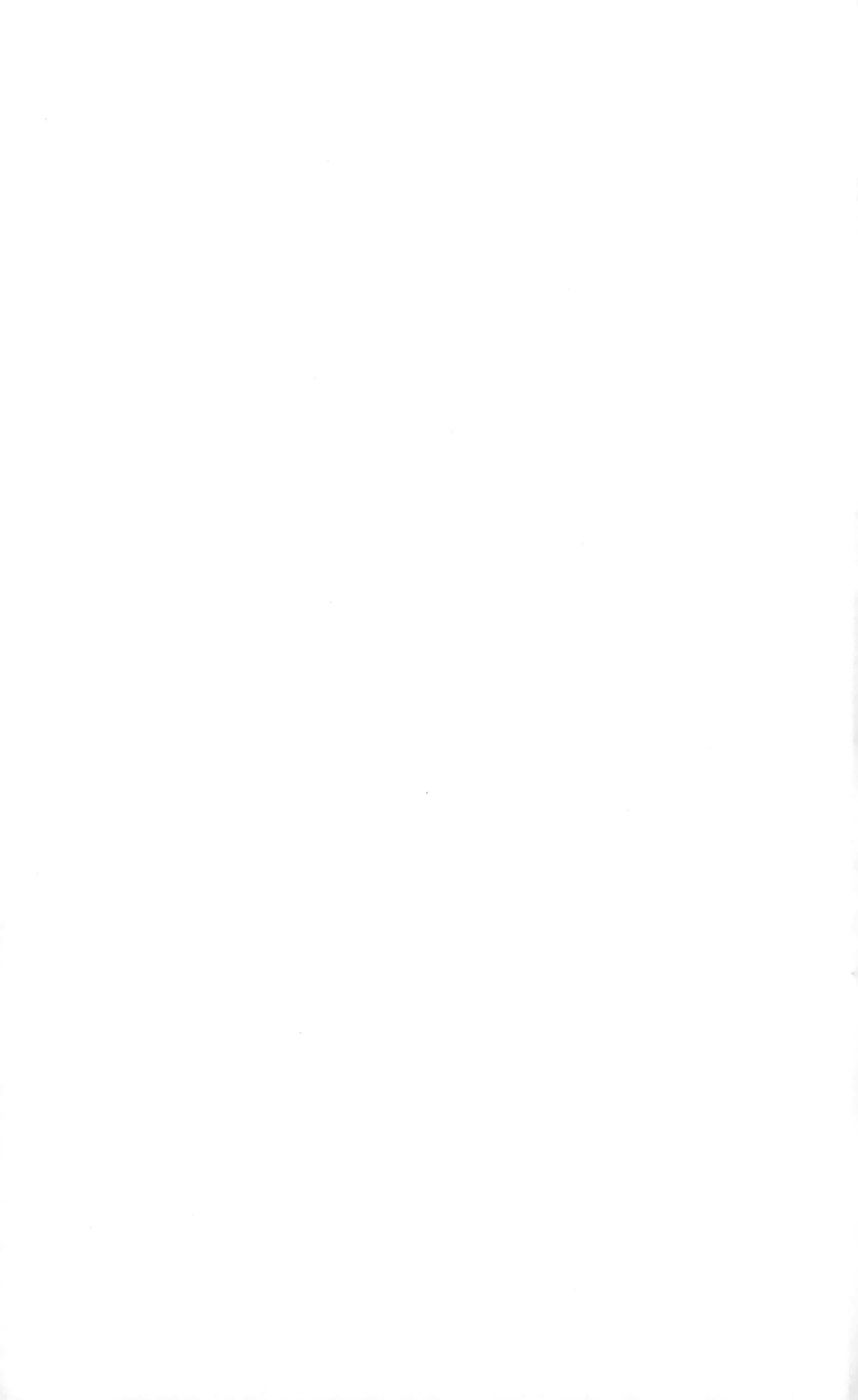

362.1
BAL
39130502
11457

Health Informatics

(formerly Computers in Health Care)

Kathryn J. Hannah Marion J. Ball
Series Editors

Springer
New York
Berlin
Heidelberg
Barcelona
Hong Kong
London
Milan
Paris
Singapore
Tokyo

Health Informatics

(formerly Computers in Health Care)

Series Editors:
Kathryn J. Hannah Marion J. Ball

Dental Informatics
Integrating Technology into the Dental Environment
L.M. Abbey and J. Zimmerman

Aspects of the Computer-based Patient Record
M.J. Ball and M.F. Collen

Performance Improvement Through Information Management
Health Care's Bridge to Success
M.J. Ball and J.V. Douglas

Strategies and Technologies for Healthcare Information
Theory into Practice
M.J. Ball, J.V. Douglas, and D.E. Garets

Nursing Informatics
Where Caring and Technology Meet, Second Edition
M.J. Ball, K.J. Hannah, S.K. Newbold, and J.V. Douglas

Healthcare Information Management Systems
A Practical Guide, Second Edition
M.J. Ball, D.W. Simborg, J.W. Albright, and J.V. Douglas

Clinical Decision Support Systems
Theory and Practice
E.S. Berner

Strategy and Architecture of Health Care Information Systems
M.K. Bourke

Information Networks for Community Health
P.F. Brennan, S.J. Schneider, and E. Tornquist

Introduction to Clinical Informatics
P. Degoulet and M. Fieschi

Patient Care Information Systems
Successful Design and Implementation
E.L. Drazen, J.B. Metzger, J.L. Ritter, and M.K. Schneider

Introduction to Nursing Informatics, Second Edition
K.J. Hannah, M.J. Ball, and M.J.A. Edwards

Computerizing Large Integrated Health Networks
The VA Success
R.M. Kolodner

Organizational Aspects of Health Informatics
Managing Technological Change
N.M. Lorenzi and R.T. Riley

(continued after Index)

Marion J. Ball   Judith V. Douglas
Editors

Performance Improvement Through Information Management

Health Care's Bridge to Success

With a Foreword by John G. King

With 14 Illustrations

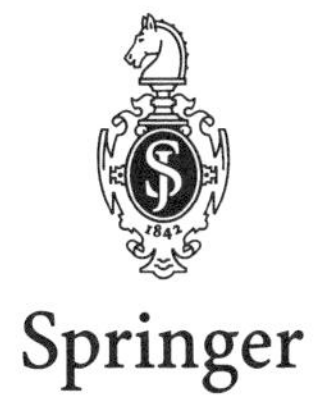

Springer

Marion J. Ball, EdD
Adjunct Professor
Johns Hopkins University School of Nursing
Baltimore, MD 21205, USA

Judith V. Douglas, MA, MHS
Adjunct Lecturer
Johns Hopkins University School of Nursing
and
Associate
First Consulting Group
Baltimore, MD 21210, USA

Series Editors:

Kathryn J. Hannah, PhD, RN
Vice President, Health Informatics
Sierra Systems Consultants, Inc.
and
Professor, Department of Community Health Science
Faculty of Medicine
The University of Calgary
Calgary, Alberta, Canada

Marion J. Ball, EdD
Adjunct Professor
Johns Hopkins University School of Nursing
Baltimore, MD, USA

Library of Congress Cataloging-in-Publication Data
Performance improvement through information management : health care's bridge to success / edited by Marion J. Ball, Judith V. Douglas.
p. cm. — (Health informatics)
Includes bibliographical references and index.
ISBN 0-387-98452-6 (alk. paper)
1. Medical informatics. 2. Health services administration.
I. Ball, Marion J. II. Douglas, Judith V. III. Series.
R858.P47 1999
362.1′068′4—dc21 98-24445

Printed on acid-free paper.

©1999 Springer-Verlag New York, Inc.
All rights reserved. This work may not be translated or copied in whole or in part without the written permission of the publisher (Springer-Verlag New York, Inc., 175 Fifth Avenue, New York, NY 10010, USA), except for brief excerpts in connection with reviews or scholarly analysis. Use in connection with any form of information storage and retrieval, electronic adaptation, computer software, or by similar or dissimilar methodology now known or hereafter developed is forbidden.
The use of general descriptive names, trade names, trademarks, etc., in this publication, even if the former are not especially identified, is not to be taken as a sign that such names, as understood by the Trade Marks and Merchandise Marks Act, may accordingly be used freely by anyone.
While the advice and information in this book are believed to be true and accurate at the date of going to press, neither the authors nor the editors nor the publisher can accept any legal responsibility for any errors or omissions that may be made. The publisher makes no warranty, express or implied, with respect to the material contained herein.

Production coordinated by WordCrafters Editorial Services, Inc., and managed by Francine McNeill; manufacturing supervised by Jeffrey Taub.
Typeset by MATRIX Publishing Services, Inc., York, PA.
Printed and bound by Maple-Vail Book Manufacturing Group, York, PA.
Printed in the United States of America.

9 8 7 6 5 4 3 2 1

ISBN 0-387-98452-6 Springer-Verlag New York Berlin Heidelberg SPIN 10663101

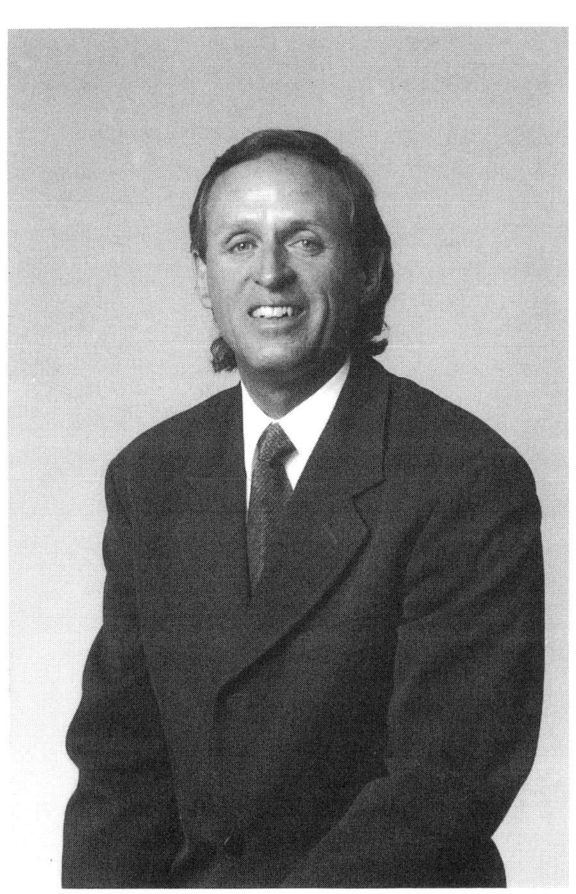

To Jim Reep, for his vision, professionalism, integrity, energy, and warmth

Foreword

Recent national surveys suggest an upturn in spending on information technology in health care and throughout corporate America. As senior healthcare executives, we cannot make these investments without justifying them in terms of what they will yield. We are charged with improving performance and delivering top-quality care. For us, buying and managing technology are only means to an end. Clearly, we have a difficult task, and we need the help of other practitioners in health care in understanding how to proceed.

To begin, performance improvement requires that we understand the forces, structures, and strategies that shape the healthcare marketplace. It demands that we change how we deliver care—that we redefine our mission and goals to prepare for the future. To achieve what we envision, we must deliberately and methodically redefine processes, restructure information, and redesign work flow.

Traditionally, efforts to improve care focus on operations at hospitals and clinics. These functions are basic to health care and assume added significance in the current environment, with its emphasis on integrating care delivery networks. Areas of fragmentation persist in health care, as do pressures to increase productivity and improve financials. Information management systems can supply critically needed linkages; increasingly robust infrastructure and applications can support integration efforts. In addition, new technologies like call centers offer innovative solutions. Clearly, we can do much to improve operational effectiveness.

The most remarkable gains in performance improvement will come from areas we are only now beginning to explore—clinical decision making for caregivers and patients alike. Today we are putting into place computerized patient records, clinical data repositories, and web-based applications. Physicians and physician managers becoming more comfortable with the technologies give them the information they need for decisions, even supply them with clinical reminders and alerts. Tomorrow, when the repositories are well populated and patient records can be confidentially shared on the web, physicians will be able to deliver care that is evidence-based, linked to the best medical knowledge.

Today, healthcare organizations are beginning to pay attention to customer satisfaction. They are collecting data, surveying patients, and offering 24-hour diala-nurse services. Real customer service offers great opportunities, largely untapped to date. For example, interactive videos can help patients share in making decisions about their treatment, and web-based modules can make patients active partners in managing their own health. For healthcare organizations, these new uses of information technology will transform health care, just as the computerized reservations process altered the airlines.

As always, the future holds risks. Fortunately, it also offcrs opportunities to those of us who understand the forces of change and seize upon transformational processes and enabling technologies to reinvent our world. To the authors of this book, who have helped us do all of these things, we offer our thanks. They have made our tasks easier.

John G. King
Chief Executive Officer
Legacy Health System
Portland, Oregon

Series Preface

This series is directed to healthcare professionals who are leading the transformation of health care by using information and knowledge. Launched in 1988 as Computers in Health Care, the series offers a broad range of titles—some addressed to specific professions such as nursing, medicine, or health administration; others to special areas of practice such as trauma or radiology. Still other books in the series focus on interdisciplinary issues such as the computer-based patient record, electronic health records, or networked healthcare systems.

Renamed Health Informatics in 1998 to reflect the rapid evolution in the discipline now known as health informatics, the series will continue to add titles that contribute to the evolution of the field. In the series, eminent experts serving as editors or authors offer their accounts of innovations in health informatics. Increasingly, these accounts go beyond hardware and software to address the role of information in influencing the transformation of healthcare delivery systems around the world. The series also will increasingly focus on "peopleware" and the organizational, behavioral, and societal changes that accompany the diffusion of information technology in health services environments.

These changes will shape health services in the next millennium. By making full and creative use of the technology to tame data and to transform information, health informatics will foster the development of the knowledge age in health care. As coeditors, we pledge to support our professional colleagues and the series readers as they share advances in the emerging and exciting field of health informatics.

Kathryn J. Hannah
Marion J. Ball

Preface

We have long believed that information technology, used wisely, can transform health care. To help make this happen, we left academia and joined the world of healthcare consulting, where we have been privileged to work with the people who effect real changes in how care is delivered. They have generously contributed their expertise to this book and to its companion volume, *Strategies and Technologies for Healthcare Information: Theory into Practice.*

This volume, *Performance Improvement Through Information Management*, presents key concepts clearly and forcefully, beginning with an insightful look at the current market environment. Subsequent chapters discuss transformational processes and enabling technologies. Throughout the volume, the focus is on making health care operationally effective by improving the processes involved in providing care and services. Information technology, our contributing authors understand, plays the role of enabler—a critical role to be sure, but always a supporting role, never the lead.

We are convinced that this new title will be an invaluable resource for chief executive officers and the entire healthcare team working to improve health care for patients worldwide. We are proud to offer this volume to our readers, new and old alike.

Marion J. Ball
Judith V. Douglas

Acknowledgments

This volume reflects the commitment and the expertise of those who contributed to it, most notably the chapter authors. Their work was supported throughout by Jim Reep, Luther Nussbaum, Philip Lohman, and Carol Moore, who helped develop the conceptual framework for the book, and Jennifer Lillis, who helped edit the pages that follow.

Other colleagues, who gave of their time to review the chapters and suggest improvements, have added richness and value to the content. Our thanks to all of the experts who serve on our review board: Homi Arabshahi, Dean Arnold, Dave Beaulieu, Marion Ball, Ray Bell, Bob Bonstein, Jim Burke, Joe Casper, Dave Chennisi, Mike Comick, John Conway, Jerry Davis, Dave Dimond, Steve Ditto, Erica Drazen, Jim Edgemon, Jim Gaddis, Hal Gilreath, Mike Gorsage, Sharon Graugnard, Kent Gray, Steve Heck, Gordon Heinrich, Barbara Hoehn, Todd Hollowell, Tom Hurley, Beth Ireton, Anna Kanski, Tom Kelly, Peter Kilbridge, Rick Kramer, Christi Liebe, Bill Looney, John Manson, Keith MacDonald, Scot McConkey, Marcia McCoy, Jim McPhail, Jane Metzger, Jeff Miller, Jerry Mourey, Mychelle Mowry, John Odden, Dave Pedersen, Leslie Perreault, Briggs Pille, Jim Porter, Nabil Qawasmi, Ted Reynolds, Keith Ryan, Debra Slye, John Stanley, Paul Steinichen, Don Tompkins, Pankaj Vashi, Tim Webb, Dale Will, Dave Williams, Roy Ziegler, and others.

Marion J. Ball
Judith V. Douglas

Contents

Part 3—Enabling Technologies

Part 1

Market Environment

1

Market Forces and the Environment

JAMES REEP AND PHILIP LOHMAN

Of all the changes to overtake health care in America since the passage of the Medicare Act in 1965, one of the least noted is the practice of referring to it *as an industry*. Earlier, we had doctors and nurses and hospitals, but no "healthcare industry" as such. What has changed, and what do the changes imply? What can we expect from the newly emerged healthcare industry? What forces will drive it, and in what direction?

What has changed is the behavior of doctors, hospitals and related providers, pharmaceutical companies, medical schools, and insurers, including government. Rather than responding autonomously to local and immediate events, they have begun to act as *groups* to address global, long-term forces and anticipate one another's responses. Because these groups offer fundamentally different products—for example, drugs and insurance—health care might not be considered an "industry" by some more exacting definitions. Yet it is an industry in the sense that it is a single enterprise involving all those who have a financial interest in sustaining human health and in curing disease. It is also organizing and restructuring itself at a pace faster than that of almost any other industry in U.S. history. With annual expenditures over $1 trillion, or almost 14 percent of the U.S. economy, it is the largest industry in the nation and, arguably, the least understood.

The healthcare industry operates in multiple environments—economic, social, technological, biological, political, and regulatory—and so is subject to a wide range of forces. Market forces, for example, are demanding lower costs and higher quality. At the same time, nonmarket forces, like the threat of antibiotic-resistant pathogens or the explosive growth of the Internet, are affecting the industry in powerful and often unpredictable ways. In combination, such forces create a volatile environment that will impose very specific conditions on any future business strategy. Our task in this chapter will be to describe these forces and analyze their impact, offer a view of the future, and sketch out the conditions we believe any successful participant strategy will have to meet.

A Snapshot of the U.S. Healthcare Market

In economic terms, health care is a good, its value realized through the marketplace activity of buyers and sellers. By definition, market efficiency is an intrinsic value, because it maximizes the relative well-being of consumers and producers. The efficiency of healthcare markets, like that of other markets, depends on three parameters: the numeric balance of participants (the number of buyers versus the number of sellers), externalities (external factors that impede or skew market functioning), and the availability of information to all participants.

By these measures, U.S. health care is a relatively inefficient and fragmented market with many monopolies and the potential for more, distortions resulting from legislative interventions, and low levels of information available to buyers. This is not the "fault" of any particular group or piece of legislation. Market participants in health care, as in other markets, simply react to the opportunities and incentives that are presented to them.

This inefficiency became evident when the rate of inflation in health care exceeded the overall rate of inflation. In the last few years, this trend reversed, as managed care became the dominant mode of healthcare financing and delivery in one geographic market after another. From its peak of 8.0 percent in 1993, the rate of change in the average healthcare benefit cost per employee fell to −1.1 percent in 1994. The rate of change rose to 2.1 percent in 1995 and 2.5 percent in 1996, but was still below the 3.0 percent overall cost inflation for those two years (Hoechst Marion Roussel 1997). Although general inflation was also falling, the decline in industry-specific inflation suggests that health care became more efficient during this period. In these few years, enrollment in health maintenance organizations (HMOs) skyrocketed from less than 30 million in 1987 to 58 million by the end of 1995 (Wilkerson, Devers, and Given 1997). Unfortunately, premiums are creeping up in some markets, as underlying costs press upwards.

Buyers and Sellers

Though hard to quantify, the balance of buyers and sellers in the healthcare market has been a factor in cost inflation. This is especially true in the acute care segment of the market, where entry barriers are high. Many smaller communities cannot support more than one hospital, leading to the creation of "natural" monopolies. Smaller communities often have the same problem with medical group practices.

Because these monopolies do not result from deliberate attempts to thwart competition, federal and state governments have only limited ability to intervene. In addition, there is a growing risk of "shared" or "administered" monopolies, as cost-driven consolidation and the drive for market share and bargaining power in the healthcare industry leave more communities with fewer health plans and a small number of more vertically integrated provider organizations (Zelman 1996).

External Factors

The healthcare market suffers from externally imposed arrangements that create friction and impede efficiency. Governments impose laws to encourage specific market behaviors; examples include medical licensing laws, the Hill-Burton Act in 1946, and the HMO Act of 1973. In some cases, special interest benefit overrides market considerations, as when a hospital or medical school is constructed to please an influential political constituency. In other cases, policymakers attempt to promote social goods despite conflicts with economic efficiency.

Another external factor that skews the demand for health care is the tax-exempt status of employer-provided healthcare benefits. Economists generally agree that employees tend to consume more health care than they would if they were paying for it directly, making them less selective consumers (Enthoven and Singer 1995). The problem is a structural one, due to the often-noted separation of the roles of buyer and consumer. The buyer, who is motivated to keep costs down, is typically not the consumer, who in theory can make cost-effective treatment choices but has little incentive to do so.

Efficiency and Information

We believe the greatest source of inefficiency has been the lack of shared information by buyers, sellers, and consumers of health care. Other things being equal, markets are efficient to the degree that buyers (employers, government, and consumers) can make informed choices and maximize the value acquired for a given price or minimize price for a given value. Consumers who pay for their own health care through copayments and deductibles often do not have enough information to make cost-effective treatment decisions even if they want to.

This lack of information makes rational decisions impossible, leads to suboptimal use of resources, and aggravates the problems created by the buyer-consumer role separation. Factors that limit information in the healthcare market include the following:

- **Complexity of medical language.** Its conceptual and theoretical structure is almost incomprehensible to buyers and consumers.
- **Fragmented structure.** Islands of information are sequestered in doctors' offices, insurance companies, hospitals, and patients' homes.
- **Absence of a national healthcare policy.** Information gathering is limited to public health, military medicine, and the aging and low-income populations covered by Medicare and Medicaid.
- **Problems of value assessment.** Quality is customarily defined in terms of resource expenditures, making independent assessments of value conceptually impossible.
- **Limited data reporting.** Experience ratings (if any) are based on insurers' disease incidence data for contract populations rather than on wellness indicators for the community at large.

- **Unavailable cost information.** The maze of factors that must be taken into account, the potentially large number of cost-bearing participants in any transaction, and the difficulty in identifying costs make it difficult to generate meaningful cost information (Luft 1997).

The healthcare market is a paradox. The United States has the world's best medical and acute care systems, leads in biomedical and biotechnology research, and produces the lion's share of the world's best medical devices and pharmaceuticals. Yet these accomplishments have not been translated into understandable value propositions for buyers and consumers. That may soon change, however, as the market undergoes rapid change.

Market Forces: Cost Control, Quality Concerns

The inefficiency of the healthcare market was tolerable to the principal buyers of health care—private employers and the federal government—as long as two conditions held. The first was that the United States enjoy competitive advantages in both foreign and domestic markets, allowing above-average investment returns and generous (and tax-deductible) expenditures on employee health, retirement, and other benefits. The second condition was that the costs of federal healthcare programs, primarily Medicare, not become large enough to pose an economic threat to the nation.

By the mid-1970s, these conditions no longer existed. Growth overseas, mainly in Japan, was threatening American control of both foreign and domestic markets in one industry after another: basic steel, consumer electronics, textiles and clothing, and machine tools. Since—according to then Chrysler chairman Lee Iacocca—the cost of employee health care in American automobiles exceeded the cost of their steel, the auto industry chose healthcare insurance as the place to start reducing labor costs. Following Chrysler's example, employers banded together in coalitions to reduce inflation in local healthcare markets by imposing limits on health insurance premiums that members would pay. The Buyers Healthcare Action Group in Minneapolis–St. Paul, the Pacific Business Group on Health, and a dozen others combined reimbursement caps with pioneering programs to increase the value of the health care they were buying.

Pressure for Cost Control

Federal attempts to control Medicare costs followed a different route: reducing utilization by changing hospital reimbursement rules. Since cost-based reimbursement created incentives for overuse and cost-report finagling by hospitals, the Health Care Financing Administration (HCFA) imposed the case-based prospective payment system (PPS). This system reimbursed hospitals not on cost of care, but on the basis of statistically derived expected cost per hospitalization. In the four years required to fully implement PPS, hospital occupancy rates plunged.

These events were a watershed. In addition to forming coalitions, employers and employer groups actively promoted specific delivery and financing arrangements: preferred provider organizations (PPOs), then point-of-service plans (POSs), carve-outs (i.e., narrowly defined, highly managed programs in areas such as mental health and substance abuse), experiments with nationwide versus regional contracting, exclusive provider organizations (EPOs), demand and disease management, direct provider contracting, and so on. Some experiments, like PPOs, have had marginal success, and employees and their unions have balked at disrupting physician relationships when employers change health plans. Still, the private sector continues to be a major source of pressure to reduce costs (Kotin and Kuhlman 1996).

There are signs that the approach larger employers take to controlling healthcare costs may change somewhat. In the short term, prosperity has lifted some pressure off the bottom line, and employers are finding that they must now compete for skilled employees who expect health insurance. In the long term, employer coalitions may become buyers of health care rather than negotiating agents for their employer members. Southern California Edison, for example, has had such a plan, called "Value 2001," under active study (Decker 1997). However, the short-term relaxation on cost control will likely disappear in the next recession, and coalitions, with their immense market power, will still be in a position to negotiate aggressively on costs.

Federal attempts to control healthcare costs have been less successful. In 1985, to address the potential bankruptcy of the Medicare Trust Fund, Congress created a "dual option" (fee-for-service and HMO) for Medicare beneficiaries. By 1991, with 49 percent of all U.S. employees under the age of 65 in a managed care plan, only 3 percent of Medicare beneficiaries were enrolled in a Medicare risk HMO, and only 6 percent were enrolled in any kind of managed care plan. Improvements to the Medicare HMO program yielded marginal results; between 1993 and 1994, Medicare enrollment in risk contracts increased by 25 percent (Zarabozo and LeMasurier 1996). Still, this amounted to just two million out of 36 million Medicare beneficiaries (*Healthcare Market Industry Yearbook* 1996).

In 1997, again reacting to predictions of a Medicare bankruptcy by 2001, Congress passed the Balanced Budget Act, including about $116.4 billion in Medicare cuts and $14.6 billion in Medicaid cuts over five years. Still, the act does not provide for changing the entitlement status of Medicare (or for any other major reform), suggesting more rounds of ever-deeper cuts if the program is to survive the rise in enrollments as members of the baby boom generation begin to retire.

Reimbursement cuts by private employers and the federal government have had a profound impact on the U.S. healthcare market. As revenues have fallen, participants in the healthcare value chain, feeling their own positions threatened, have attempted to maintain revenues and cut costs by:

- Expanding market share to achieve greater negotiating power
- Reducing staff
- Cutting utilization

- Closing, shrinking, or selling off redundant or underused facilities
- Eliminating fixed costs
- Putting increased pressure on providers of services to compete for business.

As FHP did prior to its acquisition by PacifiCare, Kaiser Health Plan has sold off a number of its hospitals and now contracts for a growing percentage of its acute care business on a competitive basis. Still, externally fixed industry revenues create a zero-sum game, where there are winners and losers. Market discipline has resulted in waves of provider and insurer consolidations.

The Demand for Quality

As long as health care was reimbursed on a fee-for-service basis and consumers had relatively unimpeded access to specialists and acute care, a high level of quality in U.S. health care was generally assumed. Though worrisome, rising costs were considered evidence of the high level of health care Americans enjoyed. The assumption was that "quality equals inputs." Each input to the system, the logic went, added value; if all the resources the physician judged necessary were placed at his or her disposal, professional skill and judgment would ensure the best possible outcome. The role of the insurer was to pay the bill and keep out of the way. Because insurers could pass on their costs and risk to employers, they made little objection.

This assumption was flawed, even dangerous. First, the reimbursement arrangements put the physician in the economically and morally anomalous position of being able to create his or her own demand, with the insurer (and, ultimately, the employer or government) paying the bill but having little influence over process or outcome. Second, the connection of resource expenditure to clinical outcomes was assumed rather than proved. Third, the belief that "more care means better care" proved to be wrong in a number of cases. Evidence of the detrimental effects of costly invasive procedures began to mount, and the high incidence of cesarean sections and other surgeries raised concern. The assumption of quality in U.S. health care begged the most important question: *Did the care people received improve their health or not?*

Concerns About Quality

Because Americans associate high levels of resource consumption and access to specialists with quality care, the reduced utilization and disrupted physician relationships accompanying managed care are triggering concerns that quality has declined as well. There are, according to Peter Boland, five specific sources of concern about healthcare quality under managed care:

- The suspicion that new reimbursement arrangements, downward pressure on utilization, and restrictions on access to care "have the potential to create hazards for patients"

- Increasing popular awareness of the variability of healthcare quality within American medicine
- The fierce competition within medical markets, where, as price competition stabilizes, participants will be expected to compete on quality
- The blurring of responsibility for quality control as clinical services are outsourced
- The "commonly held belief that quality in medical care is directly related to expenditures. The transition from cost-based reimbursement to prospective payment has heightened the perceived conflict between quality and cost" (Boland 1990, p. 422).

Concern over quality under managed care has been heightened by highly public controversies over patient dumping, reimbursement for "experimental" procedures, minimum postsurgical hospital stays, and a variety of clinical errors and omissions. As a result, there is now a consensus that quality issues must be addressed. According to Paul Ellwood, widely regarded as the "father of managed care,"

> The American health system works. It has contained costs, it provides easily accessible comprehensive health care to its insured members and, on the whole, it has not yet jeopardized quality. But patients, physicians, the uninsured and the country deserve better. The American health system is a work in progress; it can and, we believe, will get better. (Ellwood 1996, p. 1083)

Though still disorganized and diffuse, the demand for quality has become a pervasive, powerful force affecting American health care at nearly every level.

Sources of the Demand for Quality

The demand for quality in health care is coming from three principal directions: employers, government, and consumers. Employer strategy in health care has, until recently, been primarily cost-driven, aimed at holding down premiums. This is not because employers are indifferent to quality; rather, healthcare quality information has been fragmented, inaccessible, and difficult to interpret, and pressures for cost reduction have been so insistent that employers and employer coalitions have had to concentrate on cost and accept health plan assurances on quality.

This situation is changing rapidly. Although employers responding to a national survey put quality of care in fourth place (behind cost of employee and dependent care and government regulation) among their concerns in buying health care for employees, 60 percent of the respondents said they were "very concerned" about assuring quality of care (Hoechst Marion Roussel 1997). Employers are creating, or joining, a growing number of healthcare quality-oriented organizations, with a variety of goals and approaches. Some of these are:

- **National Committee for Quality Assurance (NCQA).** While the nonprofit NCQA is not an employer organization, it accredits health plans and promotes the use of the Health Employer Data Information Set (HEDIS). Under continuous development by the Committee on Performance Measurement, a consortium of employers, public buyers of health care, consumers, labor unions, health plans, and measurement experts, HEDIS is in its third release (1997) and increasingly oriented toward outcomes and consumer satisfaction. NCQA is making this information easily available in comparative format through its Quality Compass program.

- **The Foundation for Accountability (FACCT).** Founded in 1995 by Paul Ellwood, FACCT is a nonprofit consortium of healthcare buyers and consumers (HCFA, the Department of Defense, the American Association of Retired Persons (AARP), American Express, and GTE). FACCT's approach is to develop measures of care that will make health plan quality comprehensible to the consumer. So far, FACCT has released measurement protocols for such conditions as breast cancer, diabetes, depression, health risks, and health plan satisfaction. FACCT protocols are formulated to respond to consumer concerns—for example, by measuring the percentage of breast cancers diagnosed at an early stage. It is noteworthy that FACCT addresses access issues in addition to those of quality.
- **Regional or state-level healthcare quality consortia.** Largely employer-financed, many of these are using a variety of tools to obtain quality information and publish it for consumers. These include the Pacific Business Group on Health, the Buyers Healthcare Action Group in Minneapolis–St. Paul, Cleveland Health Quality Choice, the Georgia Business Forum on Health, the Tri-State Business Group on Health, and many others, some of which act as buying agents for their employer members.
- **Labor and trade unions.** The original force behind employer-provided health insurance, unions are increasingly aggressive crusaders for quality (and lower member costs) through contract negotiation with employers and, in partnership with employers, in regional healthcare councils and coalitions.

At the same time, the federal government is moving its Medicare and Medicaid beneficiaries from fee-for-service to managed care and, consequently, dealing with many of the same health plans that serve the private employer market. In the words of its administrator, Bruce Vladek, the HCFA has survived years of "setting up mostly disconnected quality hurdles for providers to jump through" (Vladek 1997), and has moved to "developing an integrated program that would make HCFA, for the first time, genuinely able to purchase services to improve the health of [its] beneficiary population." This shift will involve a good deal of program reorganization and, notably, the adoption of HEDIS 3.0 as the main tool for assessing both outcomes and member satisfaction with services.

Thus, the nation's two largest buyers of health care—private employers and the federal government—have begun to agree on a definition of healthcare quality and a common set of tools for implementing this definition.

Also demanding quality is the emerging consumer movement, which springs from a wide range of sources: the long tradition of consumer activism in the United States; the politically astute, pragmatic baby boom generation now in middle age and entering its high-utilization years (Regina Herzlinger, cited in

Hagland 1997); the anxiety and annoyance felt by many healthcare consumers (particularly union members) as they are swept up in the healthcare industry's turmoil; and a string of widely reported controversies involving HMOS, including lawsuits by disaffected members.

Consumer demands affect the healthcare industry in several ways. Consumers begin by making their desires and displeasure known to their legislators with a spate of constituent letters. Then, consumers organize. The nation has a growing and diverse population of healthcare consumer groups:

- Academically oriented organizations like the Foundation for Informed Medical Decision Making, which is affiliated with Dartmouth University
- Lobbying organizations such as the Consumer Coalition for Quality Health Care, based in Washington, D.C.
- Single-issue organizations like the new National Patient Safety Foundation
- Local groups of every stripe, many with a good deal of press savvy.

The cumulative weight of these organizations is substantial, especially when they team with employers in regional or statewide consortia to gain access to healthcare quality data. One result: in the 1997 session, the California legislature faced over 100 healthcare bills, most designed to strengthen state control of HMOs.

Consumers also vote with their feet, disenrolling from primary providers and entire health plans. This tactic is increasingly influential. As consumers get legislative and labor union support for more healthcare alternatives, their choices become more effective because more choices are made. The penalty on disfavored health plans can be severe. Not only do they lose business, they also find that the instability of revenues makes long-term planning difficult.

Consumers are taking more responsibility for their own health and health care, continuing the revolution that began in the late 1980s, when AIDS patients used the emerging Internet to explore alternative therapies and offer each other support and advice. Today, before checking into a hospital, many patients have already combed the vast electronic library, formulated questions about new medical trends and therapies, and read books like Blau and Shimberg's *How to Get Out of the Hospital Alive: A Guide to Patient Power* (1997). Though well-informed patients have the power to contribute to their own wellness, they also pose new challenges. Physicians are beginning to grapple with the unfamiliar task of defending their reasoning and decisions, and actively involved patients are becoming aware of the pioneering quality reporting programs now used by Kaiser, Voluntary Hospitals of America, Premier, and other providers and insurers. Clearly, demands for healthcare quality will become more focused and specific.

The Cost/Quality Equation

The drive to cut costs in health care is not new. What is new is the effectiveness of cost-cutting efforts and the depth of concern these efforts are provoking. Recent years have seen an influx of bold tactics designed to slash the rate of healthcare inflation; these include coalition-based buying, closed provider panels, administrative controls on utilization and capitation, group purchasing, controlled formularies, and downsizing.

Each of these tactics raises quality concerns. For example, do closed panels drive good doctors out of medicine to replace them with compliant, bottom-line-oriented "strategic partnerships"? Can a physician be expected to keep the patient's interest uppermost in mind when the cost of the authorization for specialty care will, in effect, come out of the physician's pocket? Is there a "quality floor" below which an institution simply cannot be downsized?

These questions have generated debate and provoked dozens of studies, some financed by groups with a stake in the outcome of the debate. Evidence available from study of a limited number of health plans suggests that while costs and utilization have gone down, quality of care is at least comparable to that in non-HMO environments (Luft 1997).

If implementing change is a challenge, assessing the merit of each effort is just as difficult. Research is complicated by the number of factors needing assessment and the fact that almost any answer is an attempt to hit a moving target. Managed care is changing not only how health care is reimbursed, but also who delivers it, who gets it, and how that care is given. At the same time, the evolution of medical technology is changing the content of care and cost parameters almost daily, making many comparisons less meaningful as the system evolves.

Non-Market Forces

While market forces are having a seismic effect on the U.S. healthcare industry, outside forces are having similarly pervasive effects. Changes in social policy, demographics, diseases, and advances in biomedicine and technology can change the environment drastically and unleash completely different market incentives.

Efficiency and Social Policy

After two decades of experimentation with managed care, 1993 was a watershed year. With the death of the Clinton administration's American Health Security Act in Congress, the United States was committed to an objective unique among the world's advanced economies: the creation of a true healthcare market, with healthcare providers and insurers subject to the market's tests of efficiency, within broad limits set by social policy and consensus.

The last qualification is important. While wanting lower healthcare costs and apparently permitting the market to reduce them, we as Americans do not embrace the implications of a strict market system in health care. Rather, we try to use the market to achieve both explicit economic objectives—i.e., lower costs—and implicit policy goals. As a matter of policy, we refuse to accept the condition of the market that the indigent cannot participate. Instead, we require non-profit hospitals to operate in a competitive environment and justify their tax-exempt status by providing specified levels of indigent care, and we press for-profit hospitals to do so as well, thus subsidizing care for the poor through both the tax and insurance systems. Indeed, much of the creativity and ingenuity of American health care appears along this market/policy frontier, where the industry tries to negotiate healthcare delivery arrangements that satisfy inherently competing constituencies.

Part of the creative tension between economics and social policy is being played out at the state level as federal authority is "devolved" to the states, which are being encouraged to play the role of "laboratories" where the federal role is minimized and private action encouraged. It is still too early to determine how well this strategy is working. Most state initiatives target moving Medicaid populations into various managed care arrangements, a process that is exceedingly complex.

Two long-term consequences of devolution to the states may, however, be surprising:

- The re-creation of a quasi-regulated market as voters, consumers, and some care provider groups press state legislatures to restore features of fee-for-service (e.g., mandated hospital stays, open access to specialists), enact minimum standards of care (e.g., minimum nurse staffing levels) into law, restrict a wide variety of insurance practices, and pass any-willing-provider laws.
- The standardization and integration of health care into a national (though not nationalized) industry through the imposition, by nationwide employer and industry groups, of uniform quality and reporting standards, clinical best practices, and operating policies (e.g., custody of patient information). This will be expedited by two trends: first, the accelerating consolidation of the provider and health plan segments in certain markets, a topic discussed at length in Chapter 2; second, the continuing "wiring" of health care as advanced information and telecommunications technology creates a common information platform for the industry.

These paradoxical effects of devolution may be accelerated by the potential "back-door" reentry of the federal government into the field of healthcare policy. In March 1997, President Clinton appointed an Advisory Commission on Consumer Protection and Quality in the Health Care Industry. While this commission had no legislative authority, its report, in the form of a "bill of rights" for health care, may set the tone for increased federal activism.

Three thorny issues remain. One of these, entitlement funding, has yet to be addressed. The other two are equally difficult and are built into the very structure of healthcare economics and medical science. The first is access to care. While the market provides for those who either have private insurance or qualify for government programs like Medicaid, the nation has yet to face the problem of how to care for the more than 40 million uninsured—about three quarters of them employed at low-wage jobs just above the federal poverty line—who fall between the two categories. The second is the escalating number of controversies in bioethics. In addition to the abortion debate, we now face problems raised by genetic testing, cloning, the use of fetal tissue in research and therapy, patient self-management, and physician-assisted suicide.

Demographics and Diseases

In 1996, the oldest members of the baby boom generation turned 50. Clearly, America is "graying." Today, for every 100 persons aged 18 to 64, there are 21 Americans aged 65 and older. This "dependency ratio" will hold until about 2010, when it will begin to grow, reaching 28 by 2020 and almost 36 by 2030. (Shapiro 1997). These numbers threaten the long-term stability of federal entitlement programs, including Medicare, particularly in view of the failure of either political party to address the programs' structural problems.

Moreover, many boomers have grown up with a high level of assumed autonomy and appear more inclined to take responsibility for their health than previous generations. They are also sophisticated buyers, informed about technology and unafraid to use it. While their questions and demands may feel like part of the problem, self-reliant boomers will also be part of the solution.

A less tractable problem is the uncertain public health environment ahead. The most immediate concern, of course, is AIDS—a global scourge that, in many developing countries, invites comparison with the Black Death that devastated Europe in the 14th century. One *Los Angeles Times* study (Oldham 1995) estimates that by 2000, total accumulated costs to the global economy could reach $514 billion, wiping out 1.4 percent of the world's aggregate gross domestic product.

As devastating as it is, the AIDS epidemic is only one component of what some commentators have called "the return of communicable disease." Streptococci and staphylococci are becoming resistant to a growing list of antibiotics. New diseases such as bovine spongiform encephalopathy, Legionnaires' disease, and Lyme disease are emerging, and old diseases like tuberculosis are posing new threats. Existing diseases, especially food-borne diseases like *e.coli* infections, are acquiring new virulence.

Clearly, America's healthcare industry will face challenges that will tax its material and intellectual resources to their limits. We are fortunate that the U.S. healthcare system has the scientific and organizational capabilities to deal with these issues.

The Advance of Biomedicine

One commentator has noted that while the 19th century was the golden age of physics, the late 20th century is the golden age of biology. *We suggest that it is the golden age of the application of basic science to human needs.* While the theories of evolution and natural selection had only an indirect application to medicine, biological science now progresses quickly from theory to validation to application. Genetic therapy, laser surgery, viral genomes in vaccines, cholesterol-lowering drugs, "second"-generation antibiotics, hemoglobin therapeutic "blood replacements," artificial body parts like heart valves, proteinase inhibitors—these and scores of other advances have flooded from the laboratories in the last decade. Despite reduced funding in some areas, the rate of discovery remains so high that even physicians in the narrowest subspecialties have difficulty keeping up.

Still, there are shadows in this bright picture. Many new treatments have mixed cost effects: some increase overall case costs by extending the lives of the chronically ill, some lower case costs by replacing less effective treatments, and some increase case costs simply because the increment of cost is greater than the increment of clinical effectiveness (an issue of current debate with respect to cardiac thrombolytics). Many discoveries in medical technology are applied to patients in the last stages of life, where they do not heal but merely prolong minimal biological function, a practice that a small but growing number of critics are questioning (Califano 1994).

In addition to the thorny problems of resource allocation, new technologies raise major policy questions. In particular, the success of genetic analysis in identifying genetically linked susceptibility to diseases challenges established insurance principles and threatens widespread discrimination. It has already created a storm of controversy and fostered a growing stack of legislation (National Institutes of Health 1997).

Information Technology

Starting far behind other industries, health care has undergone a forced-draft migration to automated systems over the past 10 years. Today, leading facilities in health care nearly equal those in other service industries in the use of information systems, and the average level of information automation is climbing steadily. The reason for this is simple. As the move from fee-for-service to managed care forced the industry to search for ways to cut costs, information technology was ready at hand. Its obvious targets were high labor costs of routine and often redundant clerical operations.

Much of the promise of information technology went unrealized as the healthcare industry invested in computer systems that did little more than layer automated costs on top of manual costs. Generally, the healthcare industry repeated the same mistakes other industries had made earlier—not defining stable objectives for projects and not investing in management as well as hardware and software, automating manual processes rather than redesigning them, and, above all, treating information technology as a "support" capability and therefore as peripheral to the organization's mission and strategy.

To be fair, the early failure of information technology to accomplish its widely advertised goals in health care was partly a result of the limitations of the technology of the time: slow, rigid, unstandardized, arcane, requiring legions of support technicians, and almost incomprehensible to the executives who had to pay for it and the managers, physicians, nurses, staff, and patients who had to live with it.

The situation has changed, slowly and painfully but decisively. Healthcare executives are learning from the experience of other industries and from their own mistakes. Budgets and accountability are tighter, and the technology itself is better—faster, easier to use, more forgiving, more standardized and hence more flexible, and much more powerful. Above all, the perceived role of information technology in health care has changed. Rather than being applied in piecemeal fashion to whatever routine manual processes offer themselves, information technology is being used in powerful new ways:

- To break down bureaucratic, departmentally focused organizational structures
- To create radically different, flatter, process-centered organizations
- To foster efficient and effective integration of the continuum of care. (VanEtten 1996)[1]

Indeed, it is the application of information technology to process analysis and design that has begun to compound value in health care, particularly in clinical areas. At Brigham and Women's Hospital in Boston, for example, benefits from a project to minimize adverse drug events total $4 billion when extrapolated nationwide (*Cost Reengineering Report* 1997).

In addition, the "information revolution" in health care is catalyzing the consumer movement, largely through the Internet and its support for thousands of health-related web sites (Thomasson 1997). While the healthcare marketplace has not yet become a "reverse market"—one "in which the customer, armed with a growing amount of information, uses that information to search out vendors offering the best combination of quality and price tailored to his or her individual needs" (Thomasson 1997)—it is clearly moving in that direction. The Internet is fostering not only growth but specialization (web sites devoted to eating disorders spin off web sites devoted to eating disorders of adolescents) and a proliferation of types of communities: business to business, business to consumer, consumer to consumer. With each new link, another breach is made in the walls that have kept American health care fragmented.

To succeed in its use of information technology, the healthcare industry must overcome obstacles. First, there is no single language that covers all of medicine. The Library of Medicine's Unified Medical Language System (UMLS), is still under development, as is the Health Level 7 (HL7) clinical data standard. Second, the present state of network and database technology does not assure the level of security required for clinical data in the projected applications. Third, although the recent Kennedy-Kassebaum bill offers a structure for health information confidentiality, much work remains to be done in implementing it. Fourth, despite the massive migration of Americans onto the Internet, large segments of the population remain outside the "computer revolution"—most of the poor and the aged, many of the ill. Finally, even for those who are computer-literate, information technology is often too complex, too expensive, and evolving too

---

[1]VanEtten's thesis has been widely misread: he opposes not spending on information technology, but rather the delusion that spending on systems will in itself produce value—i.e., the "input" fallacy identified earlier here with healthcare quality.

rapidly. Fortunately, for the most part, these are technical issues that lend themselves to systematic and incremental solutions. The healthcare industry's newly emerging strength in information and process management will be much in demand in coming years, which promise to be turbulent.

An Environment of Maximum Uncertainty

No longer in the protected backwater of regulation and nearly guaranteed revenues, the U.S. healthcare industry is increasingly investor-owned and a member of the mainstream market economy. Both the industry and its individual participants will have to deal with change from every direction. Still, it is a misperception to see the external forces on the industry univocally as "threats." They are, rather, opportunities to fulfill the industry's highest mission: to serve. Every new disease, every affliction, every wrenching social transformation, every burst of new technology, is a call. The issue for the U.S. healthcare industry, in its newly competitive market, is to develop the means to answer.

Conditions of Future Strategy

Since the 1980 publication of Porter's landmark book *Competitive Strategy*, discussions in the business literature have focused on defining strategy and its role, while paying much less attention to the issue of executability. This is unfortunate, since business problems reported in the press—for example, the recent sharp decline in the fortunes of HMOs ("Hit Where It Hurts" 1997)—stem from failures of execution at least as often as failures of strategic concept. Examples are legion, from IBM's problems in its belated attempt to follow Compaq down the cost curve to America Online's capacity problems as it sought to build market share. Time and again, good ideas—"gain market share to increase negotiating power"—stumble on unforeseen obstacles and failed managerial judgment. Clearly, the most basic condition of any strategy is that management be able to implement it with a reasonable chance of success. This means that strategies must be chosen and shaped with an eye to the ability of the organization to make them work successfully.

The conditions of success for any strategy might be called "metastrategies" in the classical sense in that they *precede* strategy (Chakravarthy 1997).[2] In health care, there are several "metastrategic" keys to any strategy:

- **Ability to see the source of value.** As trends gather momentum, subtle changes occur. For example, healthcare organizations, having made the conceptual shift from providing services to supporting wellness among contract populations, are beginning to see themselves as being in the business of building healthier communities.

---

[2]Chakravarthy (1997) offers a useful summary of several models of strategy, although most of his examples are taken from the information and telecommunications systems and services industry.

- **Speed.** Moving quickly is crucial to strategic execution. IBM's problem with the PC market, for example, was only one instance of a bigger problem: IBM's repeatedly late adoption of technologies and strategies that had already given its competitors the high ground. Within health care, HMOs that have moved too slowly have found themselves at a serious disadvantage in the battle for market share.
- **Value chain positioning.** The ability of an organization to reposition itself in the industry value chain allows it to take advantage of shifting industry economics. For example, downward pressure on acute care occupancy could make fixed costs an increasing and potentially unacceptable percentage of total cost. Recogition of this shift has spurred the current wave of hospital divestitures as owned-asset integrated delivery networks convert to contractual models.
- **Organizational flexibility.** The ability to translate strategy quickly into organizational structure can be decisive. An integrated delivery network that competes for global capitation had better have the ability to administer it; the physician hospital organization that wants to implement service line management will need capabilities that were unnecessary when it operated on a department-centered basis. At the same time, organizations must be able to rationalize and simplify their basic business and clinical processes to cut labor costs, shorten cycle times, and control outcomes.
- **Sustainability.** The success of a strategy depends on how well the organization can initially operationalize and subsequently sustain it. For example, an organization must be able to maintain its differentiation strategy in the face of attempts to match it. This requires sustaining a quality lead so great that either (a) its competitors cannot match it or (b) other incentives for its customers to switch to competitors are insufficient (Porter 1980).

How are these conditions to be met? For most of its history in health care, information technology has been centralized and inflexible, used to automate routine manual tasks like registering patients, collecting charges, and printing paychecks. While computers have succeeded reasonably well in this role, financial paybacks have often been elusive because the computer tended either to replace low-wage people (clerks) with higher-wage people (computer operators, systems programmers, network technicians) or, worse, simply to add another layer of costs.

Today, computers are versatile, and networks capacious and flexible. We can apply them to goals far beyond reducing the number of employees in patient accounting. We now have the technical ability to rebuild entire organizations around highly "informated" core processes, the way a sculptor uses a wire armature to build up a human figure. This means that information technology, if applied properly, can free health care of manual process bottlenecks as it has other industries. With its flexibility and power, information technology is not, in itself, a guarantee that the U.S. healthcare industry can meet the challenges that it faces; however, we believe it does provide the fundamental capability for implementing any strategy that is to have a hope of success.

The genius of free markets is the speed with which they adapt to change by altering the incentives that drive behavior. But *free markets are efficient only to the extent that their participants are individually efficient* (e.g., an obsolete steel mill reduces, through waste and pollution, the efficiency of the overall market). While we cannot do much in the short term about the externalities and policy inefficiencies built into the U.S. healthcare market (nor, in some cases, would we want to), we can increase the efficiency of the organizations we serve, and improve performance through information management.

References

Blau, Sheldon and Shimberg, Elaine Fantle. 1997. *How to Get Out of the Hospital Alive: A Guide to Patient Power.* New York: Macmillan.

Boland, P. 1990. *Making Managed Healthcare Work: A Practical Guide to Strategies and Solutions.* New York: McGraw-Hill.

Califano, J. 1994. *Radical Surgery—What's Next for American Healthcare.* New York: Times Books/Random House.

Chakravarthy, B. 1997. "A New Strategy for Coping with Turbulence." *Sloan Management Review,* Winter: 69–82.

Cost Reengineering Report. 1997. 2(10), October.

Decker, B. 1997. Manager, Healthcare and Employee Services, Southern California Edison. Conversation with author, January 22.

Ellwood, P. 1996. "Managed Care, A Work in Progress." *Journal of the American Medical Association,* October 2.

Enthoven, A. and S.J. Singer. 1995. "Market-Based Reform: What to Regulate and by Whom." *Health Affairs,* Spring: 109–119.

Hagland, M. 1997. "Focused Factories: Giving Consumers What They Want." *Healthcare Forum Journal,* September/October: 24.

Healthcare Market Industry Yearbook. 1996. Managed Care Information Center, Wall Township, N.J.

"Hit Where It Hurts—Why HMO Profits Are Shrinking Fast." 1997. *Business Week,* October 27: 42–43.

Hoechst Marion Roussel. 1997. "The State of Healthcare in America, 1997." A report of *Business and Health.* Kansas City, Mo.: Hoechst Marion Roussel, p. 4.

Kotin, A. M. and T. J. Kuhlman. 1996. "The Employer's View of Managed Care: From a Passive to an Aggressive Role," in *The Managed Health Care Handbook,* 3rd ed., ed. P. R. Kongstvedt. Gaithersburg, Md.: Aspen.

Luft, H. 1997. "Perspectives and Evidence on Efficiency in Managed Care Organizations," in *Competitive Managed Care: The Emerging Health System,* eds. J. D. Wilkerson et al. San Francisco: Jossey-Bass, pp. 41f.

National Institutes of Health. 1997. "Genetic Testing for Cystic Fibrosis." NIH Consenus Statement Online. April: 14–16 (especially Section 4).

Oldham, J. 1995 (October 13). The Economic Cos of AIDS." *Los Angeles Times.*

Porter, M. 1980. *Competitive Strategy.* New York: Free Press.

Porter, M. 1985. *Competitive Advantage.* New York: Free Press.

Shapiro, D. 1997. "Fluctuating Fertility: The Baby Boom and the Baby Bust." Department of Economics, Pennsylvania State University, Spring.

Thomasson, W.A. 1997. "Wellness on the Net," in *1998 Guide to Health Care Resources on the Internet*, ed. John Hoben. New York: Faulkner and Gray.

VanEtten, P. 1996. "Spend More, Get Less." *Healthcare Forum Journal*, November/December: 34.

Vladek, B. 1997. "HCFA's Quality Improvement Program" [speech transcript]. http://www.hcfa.gov, October 15.

Wilkerson, J.D., K.J. Devers, and R.S. Given. 1997. "The Emerging Managed Care Marketplace." *Competitive Managed Care: The Emerging Health Care System*. San Francisco: Jossey-Bass.

Zarabozo, C. and J.D. LeMasurier. 1996. "Medicare and Managed Care," in *The Managed Health Care Handbook,* 3rd ed., ed. Peter R. Kongstvedt. Gaithersburg, Md.: Aspen, p. 703.

Zelman, W.A. 1996. *The Changing Healthcare Marketplace*. San Francisco: Jossey-Bass.

2

Market Structure

Roice D. Luke and Ramesh K. Shukla

There is little doubt that the healthcare industry continues to undergo major and rapid change. However, there is considerable uncertainty as to what kinds of organizations will remain once the restructuring of markets has run its course. Will hospital firms move into powerful vertical systems, or stop at the safer shores of horizontal combinations? Will physicians align with hospitals locally, or opt to join up with national physician practice management companies? Will managed care companies align with integrated systems, or seek to divide and conquer at the local market level?

In this chapter, we examine the structure of healthcare markets in three steps. First, using an economic framework for assessing market competition, we pinpoint some important strategic battles in the healthcare industry. Then, we discuss the primary structural features of the markets, assessing the intensity of competition for three important healthcare sectors: managed care, hospital systems, and physician groups. Lastly, we review the idea, widely accepted in the healthcare industry, that the restructuring of markets is sequential, predictable, and moving toward some final market stage.

Economic Model and Strategic Battles

In his widely recognized model, Porter introduced a framework identifying the interplay between the major competitive forces within markets (1980). As shown in Figure 2.1, five key threats drive competition within most markets. These stem from possible entrants, buyers, sellers, substitutes, and rivals. In our analysis, the category of rivals equates to the provider sector. For example, when examining hospital markets, we place hospitals and hospital systems in the "rival" box, make insurers the buyers, and so on. Importantly, we note that the intensity of threat emanating from each sector varies across the five and over time.

Because our interest is ultimately in provider systems, we break out physician from hospital competitors. Of course, there is much cooperation between these two, but the competitive struggles between them is emerging as one of the major battles in health care. Two other battles are also taking shape—one between

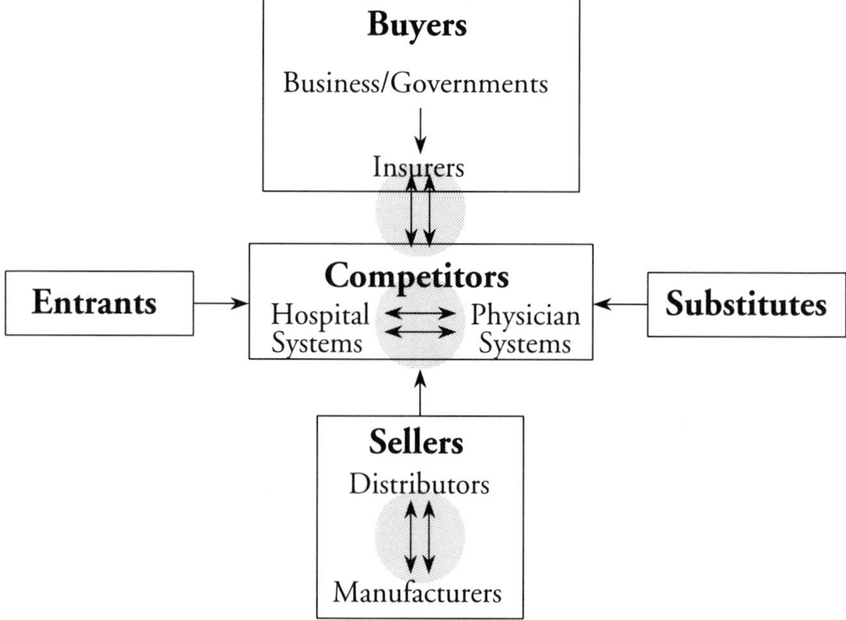

FIGURE 2.1. Structure: Assessing Sources of Market Threat and Opportunity

providers and insurers for control over the channels for distributing health insurance, and one between distributors and manufacturers over control of the restructuring supply-distribution channels. Each of the three battles is highlighted in Figure 2.1 and discussed briefly below.

Hotspot 1: Hospitals versus Physicians

The struggle to control integrated delivery has the potential to erupt into war between local hospital systems and physician organizations. Granted, the hospital sector is already highly consolidated at the local level, while the physician sector lags far behind in terms of local consolidation. This gives hospital systems the lead in forming integrated systems in nearly every market nationwide. However, there are exceptions that serve notice on hospital systems.

For example, large, geographically dispersed physician groups have emerged as major players in southern California, for the most part eclipsing hospital systems in the region (e.g., see Penner 1997). Physician groups have consolidated, as evidenced by the acquisition by MedPartners of some of the largest groups in the Los Angeles area. These groups also are major players in Minneapolis, arguably one of the most advanced markets in the country, and elsewhere. Witness their role historically in forming physician-based systems like Henry Ford in Detroit, the Mayo Clinic, the Cleveland Clinic, and Virginia Mason in Seattle.

Can physicians in other markets create delivery organizations with enough leverage to overpower well-established hospital systems? We believe there are reasons for doubt. Because physicians in most markets are highly fragmented, they would need time to reach the requisite level of consolidation. Moreover, they would have to overcome a host of local factors, including referral structures, patterns of hospital affiliations, and resistance from individual physicians and medical groups. Any or all of these can have the power to splinter physician alliances.

Further complicating the situation are strategic deficits faced by physicians as a whole, notably the shortage of trained and experienced management talent and the lack of capital. These are not insurmountable. Many physicians are entering health administration and MBA programs to obtain formal training, while others are assuming leadership roles in provider and managed care organizations across the country. With ready access to capital, rapidly growing physician practice management companies (PPMCs) could provide corporate backup (Robinson and Casalino 1995). On the other hand, they still represent only 2 to 6 percent of the nation's physicians (Burns and Robinson 1997). Large, loosely coupled physician networks and independent practice associations (IPAs) could provide the foundation for physician-based systems, but they are more likely to remain contracting agents for community physicians. In the short term, at least, they are not likely to emerge as shapers of integrated delivery.

Finally, hospital-based systems could coopt physicians—or themselves be coopted by physicians—and bring medical staff members into leadership positions, acquire physician practices, and form physician hospital organizations (PHOs). Success here, however, would depend upon aligning incentives, sharing power, and adjusting corporate cultures to fit the special needs of physicians—a tall order.

Two alternative outcomes are possible as the battle within the provider sector winds down. In the first, either hospital systems or physician groups emerge as clear winners, with the power to form and control integrated systems. A winner could be in a position to challenge insurers for control of the distribution channels that lead to the ultimate buyers of care. In the second scenario, there is no clear winner, resulting in a relatively fragmented market environment where no one is particularly dominant. Here, the insurers could gain the upper hand by contracting selectively and with impunity with any or all of the providers in the markets.

Hotspot 2: Insurers versus Providers

This leads us to the clash between provider and insurer players, which centers on whether or not a middleman is needed. Increasingly organized as managed care organizations, insurers function as intermediaries to facilitate the distribution of health insurance products to the ultimate buyers—namely, business and industry, governments, and individuals. The battle takes several forms, including threats of either backward or forward vertical integration. Indeed, it has been one of the important early assumptions of the so-called 1990s paradigm shift that such vertical integration would occur. To the extent that it does, *it will be important to determine which sector will likely initiate vertical integration, and which will dominate the resulting structures.*

The integration of these two sectors can take the form of mergers and acquisitions or internal investments in capacity, initiated from either side. While there are examples of both approaches, the results thus far are mixed. Well-known failures include Columbia/HCA's attempt to acquire Blue Cross of Ohio and Prudential's strategy of acquiring physician practices. The first of these was never culminated, and the second has almost completely unraveled.

There are also important examples of internal expansions. Backward, internal integration by insurers into provider sectors is unlikely, if only because there is little room in any market for added provider capacity. There are, however, high-profile and apparently successful hospital players forward-integrating (internally) into managed care—for example, Sentara in Norfolk, Virginia; Sisters of Providence in Seattle; and Intermountain Healthcare in Salt Lake City.

One strategy pursued primarily by hospital systems is going directly to the buyers and eliminating the insurer middleman. This strategy is strengthened by the backlash against managed care, creating a new environment where providers may be able to position themselves as the alternative to excessive third-party intrusions. Preferred provider organizations (PPOs), provider networks, and other combinations of providers at the local level are entering the fray on two fronts—the marketplace itself and the halls of state legislatures and the U.S. Congress. Providers are pushing legislation to support the direct marketing of provider products to the buyers. If successful, this strategy threatens the very existence of the insurance industry. Still, it is unlikely that the insurers will willingly fade into oblivion. We can expect powerful countermoves if this movement gathers steam.

Today the battle between providers and insurers is at a stalemate, largely because of the limitations to vertical integration. Yet this "cold war" could easily break out into heated conflict over the control of health insurance channels. When or whether this happens will depend on developments in state and federal legislatures, consumer attitudes about managed care, and the restructuring of the markets themselves.

Hotspot 3: Distributors versus Manufacturers

A third point of intersector rivalry arises over channels for distributing healthcare supplies to providers. So far, the sellers (manufacturers and distributors) pose little strategic threat to providers. On the other hand, through creative forms of collaboration, they could offer significant competitive advantages to individual providers. The question is, which will be better positioned to do this—the distributors or the manufacturers?

The recent formation of complex delivery systems has created new opportunities to gain economies in the management of internal systems, by coordinating among the combined provider members. The distributors noted this potential early and have responded by offering a variety of collaborative arrangements through which they help provider systems improve their control over supply acquisition, product handling, inventory, and utilization (CSC Consulting 1996). As a consequence, distributors have gained increased control over the distribution channels, a development that has the potential of choking off direct access by manufacturers (pharmaceutical, medical/surgical, and other) to provider clients.

Recent years have seen dramatic moves among distributors—the spinoff of Baxter's medical/surgical distribution capability, forming Allegiance; the acquisition of General Medical (the third largest medical/surgical distributor) by McKesson (the lead pharmaceutical distributor at that point); and the attempted merger between Cardinal (pharmaceutical distribution) and Bergen Brunswig (primarily pharmaceutical but also holding an important position in medical /surgical distribution), which was stopped by the Federal Trade Commission in 1998. Undertaken for different reasons, each move highlights the changing economics within the distribution business.

Two strategies appear to be behind the restructuring in the pharmaceutical industry. The first, which responds to the forming integrated systems and overall consolidation in the healthcare industry, is to integrate across products (medical/surgical, pharmaceutical, durable products, etc.) and offer "one-stop shopping" to the forming provider systems. Information systems are key here, as it is the electronic highway that facilitates control over product handling, ordering, and inventory. The second strategy is to enter into diverse product channels (acute care, primary care, home health, long-term care, etc.). Both of these options are enhanced by the mergers and acquisitions within and across the distribution industry. All of this threatens the manufacturers who, as a result, are increasingly dependent on the distributors for access to providers. The suppliers are thus faced with the choice of working through the distributors or seeking independent channels through which they can distribute their products to their customers.

One alternative is for the forming provider systems to handle the supply functions internally. For example, Sentara Health System in Norfolk is attempting to bypass the distributors by managing its internal "redistribution" itself and working directly with manufacturers. Only a few systems are pursuing this option. More have opted to collaborate with the distributors (e.g., Kaiser of California), which, in effect, involves an outsourcing approach to the redistribution of supplies at the local level.

The upshot? Manufacturers now must weigh the implications of the restructuring channels for their long-term viability. This could lead to some interesting consolidations and perhaps countermoves in order for them to be assured independent access to their buyers. They could reassess their relationships with the distributors, possibly entering into strategic alignments with them or, somewhat less likely, moving to reclaim control over the distribution channels (e.g., Abbott's insistence on distributing its own products wherever possible) through forward integration strategies.

Structural Features

According to the industrial organization framework presented in Chapter 3, the characteristics of the markets play a major role in shaping the strategies of competitors. Of a number of structural indicators, three are among the most important:

- **Market concentration**—the degree to which the numbers of competitors and/or buyers have reduced to but a few
- **Entry barriers**—the difficulties encountered by potential new competitors as they consider entering markets
- **Product differentiation**—the degree to which individual competitors are able to distinguish themselves from one another in ways that are valued by consumers.

In general, *the more concentrated the markets, the higher the entry barriers, and the greater the product differentiation, the less likely it is that competitors will engage in behaviors that reduce or even slow increases in prices.* This does not necessarily mean that competition goes away. In markets with high concentration and few competitors (technically known as *oligopolistically* structured markets), competitors are often highly rivalrous, even if not particularly focused on price competition. Because of small numbers, such competitors tend to be very interdependent—they carefully monitor and react to each other's strategic moves. In health care, this market structure is characteristic of managed care and hospital markets, many of which have already achieved high levels of concentration. It also could eventually characterize physician markets, if trends toward consolidation continue.

Competitiveness, of course, can be stimulated by threats from other sources, as indicated in Porter's framework. The managed competition model posits strengthened buyers who aggressively stimulate price competition among managed care firms and providers. Even now, state governments, large private firms, and other buyers representing large numbers of beneficiaries exercise considerable purchasing power in local and national healthcare markets. Still, most buyers are very small and need to strengthen their positions by combining into larger buyer groups (e.g., business coalitions). Only then can they counter the rising monopolistic power of managed care firms and provider systems.

What is happening on the buyer side in health care? The much-heralded threat from buyers has fallen far short of expectations. State buyers have become mired in the politics and economics of local health care. Some have taken steps to restructure their Medicaid programs and to tinker with other policy issues. But with the possible exception of California, they have done little to take advantage of their role as major buyers within their markets. The same is true of the private sector. Since the early 1990s, many large firms have lost momentum as purchasers of health plans, probably as a result of the precipitous slowing in the rise in healthcare prices. Nor have business coalitions performed as anticipated. So far, less than a third of the Metropolitan Statistical Areas (MSAs) have business coalitions. Some of these have closed and, of those still active, only about half have evolved buyer cooperatives. Of these, barely a handful represent sufficient numbers of employees/lives to have any major impact on their markets.

If healthcare costs begin to rise again, we can expect more developments on the buyer side. Until that happens, the strategies of healthcare organizations will likely be influenced by developments within the healthcare markets themselves and the structures emerging within three major sectors—managed care, hospitals, and physicians.

Managed Care

Of the many changes in managed care during the 1990s, one of the most important is the penetration of private/commercial managed care within urban markets, which increased from 6 percent in 1982 to 27 percent as of July 1996 (InterStudy 1997). The latter was up nearly five points from a year earlier, reflecting continued strong growth in this sector.

The actual distribution in penetration across markets varies strongly by both market size and region. Table 2.1 summarizes the penetration rates for all 321 MSAs in the United States by three population size categories and four geographic regions. As the table illustrates, the greatest levels of penetration are in the largest population markets and in the West. The lowest percentages are in the smallest markets and in the South.

In addition, levels of Medicare and Medicaid managed care penetration have increased rapidly (Lamphere et al. 1997). When levels of public and private pen-

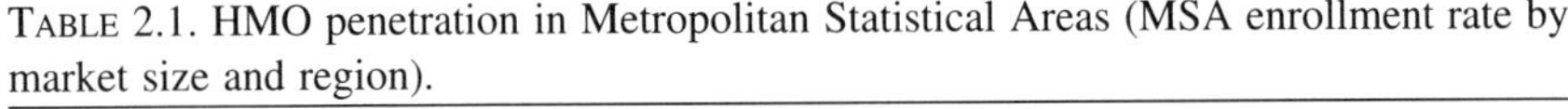
TABLE 2.1. HMO penetration in Metropolitan Statistical Areas (MSA enrollment rate by market size and region).

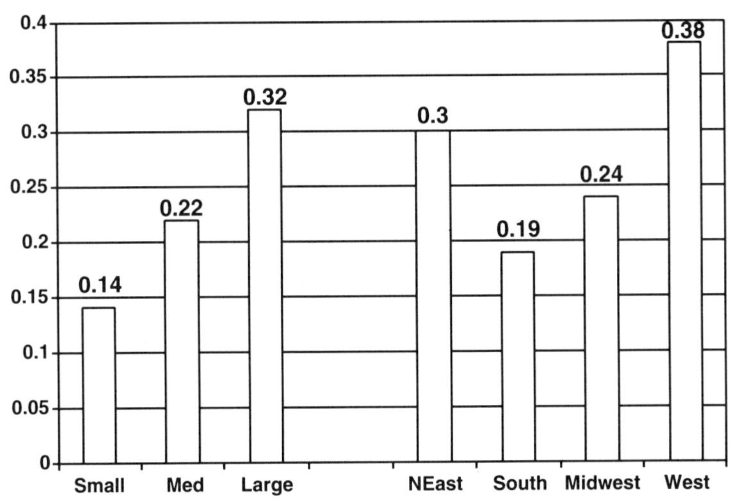

etration are combined, estimates are that just over 30 percent of the urban population are enrolled in managed care plans (InterStudy 1997). These penetration rates do not, of course, mean that capitated payment is also widespread. While precise data are unavailable, diversity in payment methods and HMO products is the rule. As Gabel has noted, most current health maintenance organizations (HMOs) "do not view themselves as HMOs, but as managed care organizations that offer an array of managed care products" (1997, p. 135).

This is an important distinction, because capitation is such a powerful tool for stimulating cost restraint among providers. The same is true for patient channeling through single signatures, which also has not kept pace with managed care penetration. Difficulties inherent in vertical integration, resistance by providers, and consumer preferences for provider choice have played major roles in defeating widespread adoption of many features essential to the managed care model.

As the markets mature, however, both capitation and channeling might yet increase, though considerable fragmentation and diversity should remain as well. Of course, all bets are off once legislation enables provider systems to direct contract and form so-called provider service organizations (PSOs). On one hand, this could have little impact, as providers come face-to-face with myriad challenges inherent in managing care and competing in an industry in which they lack experience and know-how. On the other hand, it could lead to a major restructuring of the relationships between providers and managed care firms. For example, the threat of PSOs could lead both providers and insurers to enter into more strategic collaborative arrangements (e.g., franchising by national managed care firms) at the local level.

Consolidation

Consolidation among managed care companies has grown steadily in the 1990s. By 1996, an estimated 25 companies—about five percent of managed care organizations—accounted for two-thirds of national enrollment in managed care (Gabel 1997, p. 138). Many national managed care organizations have grown very large by acquiring other HMOs. Two notable examples are the acquisition of FHP International by PacifiCare and the merger between U.S. Healthcare and Aetna. While such acquisitions lead to further consolidation at the local market level, the effects on local concentration rates thus far are minimal (Christianson, Feldman, and Wholey 1997).

Complementing the trend toward national consolidation is a movement toward for-profit status, which appears to be motivated by needs for capital to finance market growth strategies. Today, nearly 60 percent of HMO enrollment is in for-profit organizations, whereas in the late 1980s the majority of the enrolled population was in not-for-profit HMOs. This trend has impacted both commercial and Blue Cross companies.

We suspect consolidation at the local market level may prove to be even more significant. It is widely expected that three to four managed care players will dominate most local markets. The level of consolidation within markets is often measured by the Herfindahl Index, which represents the sum of squared shares among all players in a market. (Note that a market with six equally sized competitors would get a Herfindahl score of .17 and one with four equally sized competitors would receive a score of .25, meaning that markets with scores approaching or exceeding these levels are becoming highly concentrated.)

Scores calculated using 1996 data for population size categories and regions are shown in Table 2.2. All scores are .24 or higher. As expected, they vary inversely with the size of the markets, though they are fairly similar across the four regions. The scores have reached very high levels in the smaller markets, where limited populations generally result in fewer players. Scores for 1996 increased an average of .066 points over 1995—a pattern strikingly similar to that in hospital markets (see below).

Entry Barriers

Data with which to measure the height of the entry barriers are scanty. Anecdotal reports and observations of the field confirm that managed care markets remain highly contestable. New national firms regularly enter new markets, either as new entrants or by acquisition or merger. Local and regional players are forming and expanding into new markets. Although entry barriers in this sector appear fairly low now, they may change over time. Continued consolidation may foreshadow a raising of entry barriers both nationally and locally.

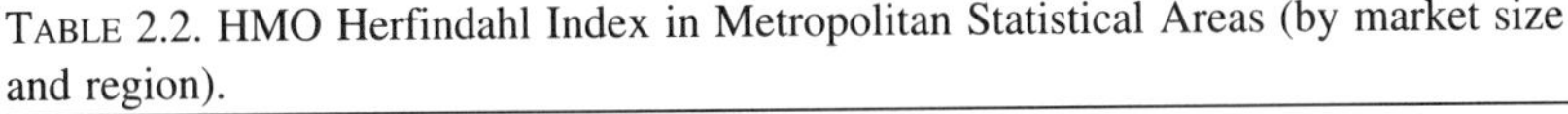

TABLE 2.2. HMO Herfindahl Index in Metropolitan Statistical Areas (by market size and region).

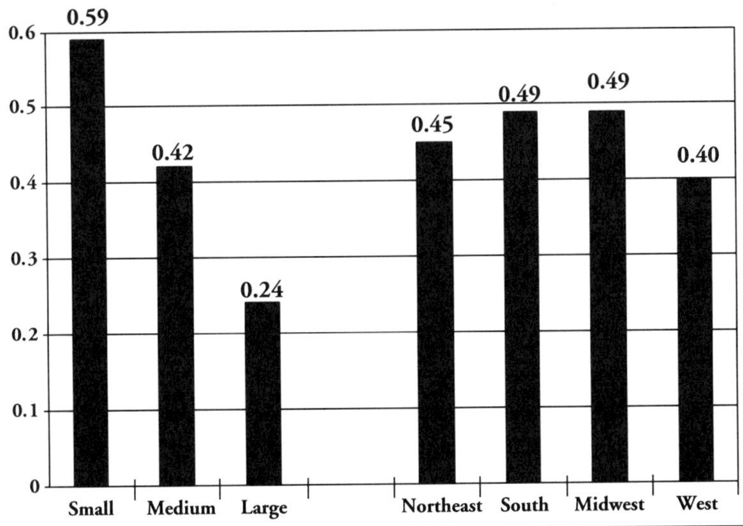

Product Differentiation

Trends in product differentiation are mixed. There has been growth in some of the newer product forms—point-of-service (POS), PPO, IPAs, and other loosely structured and mixed organizational types. Yet these products tend to be offered by all major managed care companies as they attempt to capture changing demand and gain economies. Such "copycat" behavior reduces overall levels of product differentiation across competitors.

Also, since the more open structures of the HMO products lead to broader provider networks and contracts, the insurance competitors tend to look even more alike (they have no distinctive provider arrangements to sell in their markets). These trends also have important implications for the forming integrated systems, predicated as they are on their ability to offer distinctive provider combinations.

Summary

Overall, changes within managed care appear to be having mixed effects. Steady rises in consolidation tend to reduce price competitiveness, but not levels of rivalry in general. On the other hand, moderate entry barriers and limited product differentiation contribute to price competitiveness and overall levels of rivalry. As competitors develop and refine their offerings in a process known as *commodization*, the likelihood increases that price will become a major consideration in choosing health plans. This raises one key question: *Will managed care companies over time be able to force price concessions by providers?*

As consolidation reaches its limits and pressures to control costs heighten, perhaps managed care companies will look more favorably upon vertical arrangements with providers. Doing so might allow them to capture economies of scale and improve coordination, as well as improve market positions. Beneficiaries still willing to pay a premium for provider choice could resist, but if the plans tighten relationships with selected providers, these beneficiaries may lose the leverage they now have to pick and choose among local providers and delivery systems.

In sum, the managed care markets are still very fluid and competitive. They are contestable, even with high levels of national and local consolidation, given low to moderate entry barriers and diminishing levels of product differentiation across plans.

Hospital Systems

Hospital markets are also changing, but the results could differ greatly from those in the managed care sector. For simplicity, we examine only general medical/surgical hospitals, of which there are a total of 5,114 nationally. These represent 53 percent of the total number of hospitals and 80 percent of hospital beds in the United States. Of these hospitals, 2,734 are located within MSAs. Importantly, in most markets (both urban and nonurban), the acute care general hospitals are taking the lead in system formation.

Like managed care, hospital markets are consolidating rapidly. Unlike managed care, however, the consolidation is occurring locally, not nationally. Columbia/HCA, the largest hospital firm until recent spinoffs, controlled about 6 percent of the overall urban acute care business. Other than Columbia, only a few systems have the potential to mount any kind of a national strategy (e.g., Tenet), and they are unlikely to do so.

Even without national consolidation, there has been a significant increase in hospitals belonging to systems having two or more hospitals. We call these *multihospital systems* (MHSs). By 1997, 53 percent of all general medical/surgical hospitals and 62 percent of bed capacity were in MHSs (Williamson Institute 1997). Still, the local level is where the real consolidation is taking place. In the MSAs, for example, MHS membership is very high, involving 63 percent of urban hospitals and 67 percent of beds (Williamson Institute 1997).

In addition, hospitals have combined into locally configured strategic arrangements including tighter MHS combinations and looser partnerships and joint ventures. Within MSAs, 85 percent of the hospitals in local strategic combinations are members of MHSs. Put in other terms, 78 percent of MHS urban hospitals are in some kind of strategic alignment locally, compared to only 23 percent of nonsystem (freestanding) hospitals. The primary reason hospitals join with others in local markets is to compete from positions of strength for managed care contracts and to defend against other competitor combinations. Thus, we label all such combinations of two or more hospitals *strategic hospital alliances* (SHAs).

In all, 58 percent of urban hospitals and 65 percent of urban beds are combined into SHAs. These percentages have grown steadily, increasing from 18 percent in 1982 to 29 percent in 1989 and to 58 percent in 1997. The distributions of SHA hospitals by market size and region are summarized in Table 2.3. Just as with managed care, the percentages vary strongly and directly with market size, but only slightly with region. Significantly, 65 percent of urban hospital bed capacity is joined within SHAs, reflecting the fact that larger hospitals are more likely than smaller ones to be members of strategic hospital alliances.

Consolidation

A more telling way to look at the market effects of SHAs is to examine their impact on market concentration. Tables 2.4 and 2.5 summarize market concentration using two different measures. The first (Table 2.4) is the Herfindahl Index, or the sum of squared shares among all players in a market, explained earlier in this chapter. Interestingly, the Herfindahl scores for hospitals are similar in level and pattern to those for managed care. The second measure (Table 2.5) identifies the total share controlled by the top four hospital firms within a market, where the firms can be either SHAs or freestanding hospitals.

This so-called four-firm share measure tells a powerful story about hospital consolidation. In the smaller markets (representing 48 percent of the MSAs but only 28 percent of the total U.S. MSA population), the top four firms average 100 percent of the total shares, measured in terms of hospital acute care patient

TABLE 2.3. Strategic hospital alliance penetration in Metropolitan Statistical Areas (percentage of MSA beds by market size and region).

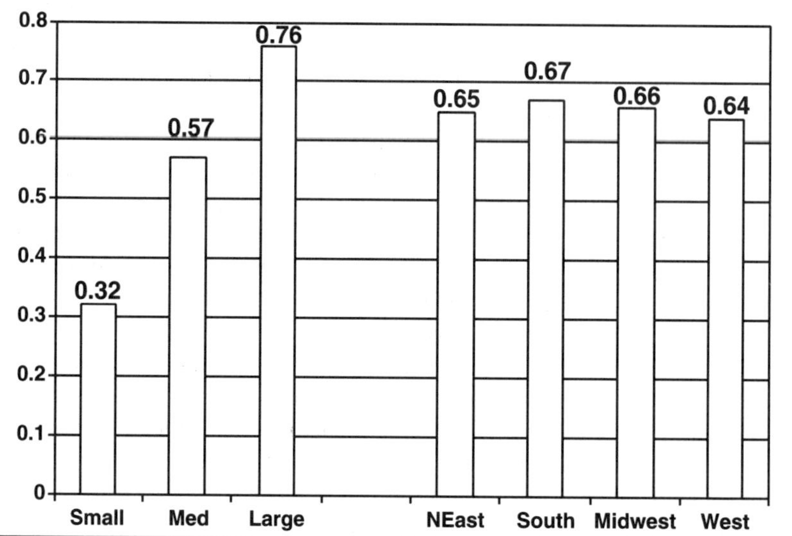

days. In these markets, which characteristically have very few hospitals or hospitals consolidated into SHAs, the top four firms easily capture fully the local markets. In the midsize and large markets (only 18 percent of all MSAs but 62 percent of the total U.S. MSA population), the percentages are 96 and 79, respectively. In many of the largest markets—Denver, Cleveland, Orlando, Tampa Bay, Fort Lauderdale, and St. Louis—the four-firm shares exceed 90 percent. In

TABLE 2.4. Hospital competitor Herfindahl Index in Metropolitan Statistical Areas (by market size and region).

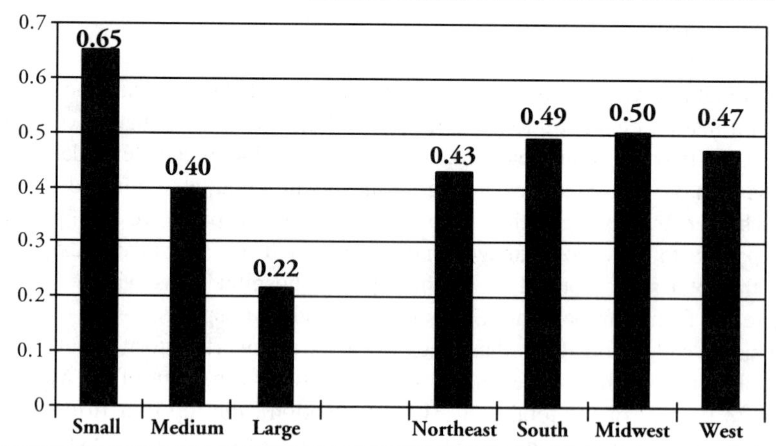

TABLE 2.5. Four-firm ratio in Metropolitan Statistical Areas (by market size and region).

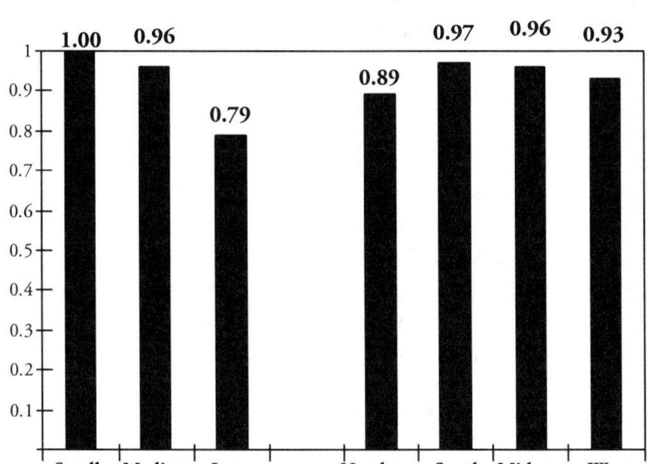

some of these markets, however, the four-firm ratios range around 50 percent and below (e.g., Philadelphia, Chicago, Los Angeles, and New York). The percentages vary slightly by region, with markets in the South having the highest average four-firm market shares and those in Northeast the lowest. Still, they are very high for all regions overall. Both measures show that the hospital markets are already very consolidated. Moreover, observation tells us that hospitals are continuing to combine in many markets.

Entry Barriers

Compared to barriers in managed care, entry barriers in hospital markets are high and getting higher. Many markets are effectively closed. Some face state restrictions against entry by capacity expansion. Others find entry by acquisition or merger is constrained, due either to resistance from established local hospitals and hospital systems or diversity and consequent incompatibilities between the suitors and their potential partners in such areas as ownership types, values, and missions. Mergers and alliance building can also be inhibited by rivalries between different types of hospitals: teaching versus community, public versus private.

Until 1997 and the withdrawal of Columbia's national strategy, many hospitals feared entry by a national system. In retrospect, their anxiety was misplaced. Today, entry from outside appears even more remote. Although there may still be movement regionally as local players combine across markets to form statewide and regional systems, entry barriers for hospital markets must be considered very high, at least for the present. As regional combinations continue, it is possible that a new wave of national system formation could be unleashed. For now, however, that prospect appears slim.

Product Differentiation

Here, the cliché "health care is local" comes most strongly into play. Hospitals and other providers enjoy relatively high levels of product differentiation. They differ in their product mixes, missions, and other essential features. Many have unique locations and loyal medical staffs who enjoy reliable referral relationships with primary care physicians, either informal or structured by managed care or network arrangements.

Such characteristics vary from hospital to hospital and system to system. In the denser urban areas, many hospitals share the same geography and therefore have no particular advantages due to location. In Houston, for example, a number of major hospitals are located within the renowned Texas Medical Center, probably the largest conglomeration of healthcare capacity anywhere in the world. Other smaller clusters exist in most major markets nationwide.

To the extent that managed care channels patients to providers, location and other differentiating features should decline in importance. However, as discussed above, channeling has yet to become widespread. Also, some markets are divided into distinctive territories, providing hospital competitors unassailable strategic niches. In Phoenix, for example, a number of geographic areas (e.g., Scottsdale, Tempe, Sun City) are controlled by individual systems and/or hospitals, making these competitors relatively impervious to threats from managed care or hospital rivals.

As discussed in Chapter 3, product quality, despite its importance in this industry, has not yet emerged as a major basis for product differentiation. There are, of course, some notable exceptions (principally, some academic medical centers and prominent institutions within selected markets across the country, e.g., the Mayo Clinic). In general, however, hospitals and especially hospital systems have not found the key to differentiation on the basis of quality. Branding also has not found a foothold in this industry. Indeed, there are some conspicuous examples where branding has failed (e.g., see the efforts of the Humana hospital system, Columbia/HCA, and other for-profit systems). As systems and strategic alliances continue to form and mature, it is probable that product differentiation will increase in this industry. To the extent that direct contracting reaches its potential, competitors will very likely turn to product differentiation to gain competitive advantage.

Summary

Of all the healthcare sectors, hospital markets are probably the most consolidated locally. The degree of consolidation, combined with very high entry barriers and relatively high levels of product differentiation, means that local hospital competition over time could be somewhat less focused on price competition than many have predicted. This does not mean that these markets will be tranquil. Local hospital markets should remain rivalrous for some time, because of high levels of interdependencies among hospitals and systems, the lingering threat of vertical integration, continuing threats from powerful managed care and physician competitors, and the prospect that direct contracting will introduce unknown market forces into this industry.

For the hospital sector, two major questions remain. First, will hospitals be successful in building comprehensive integrated delivery systems at the local market level? We believe many will be successful in consolidating horizontally, and some will succeed in integrating vertically. Second, will they pursue vertical integration into managed care or strategic alignment with managed care firms? While less likely, this may depend on developments in the area of direct contracting.

For vertical integration to become a major trend, hospital competitors would have to be capable of competing against nationally distributed managed care companies. For this to happen, hospitals themselves would have to consolidate nationally—an improbable scenario, at least in the short term. They would risk competing with their primary customers, from whom they could expect some unpleasant countervailing responses. In addition, they would be entering high up on the learning curve of a complex and quickly maturing business—a real disadvantage, given the aggressiveness and rapidity of change within the managed care sector. In time, of course, as the industry matures and direct contracting introduces further instability into the industry, the managed care and provider sectors could be brought closer by vertical integration, franchising, and other emerging strategies.

We also predict that provider systems already vertically integrated into managed care will in time sell off their managed care businesses. They will do so for two reasons: to protect themselves against strong managed care competitors, and to ensure that their own managed care businesses are not hobbled by the exigencies of local hospital system strategies. We recall Humana's failed attempt to combine hospital and managed care businesses in the 1980s. They discovered that the strategic issues facing managed care businesses differ greatly from those of provider systems.

Physician Groups

Without a doubt, the medical profession is in a position to control the whole of health care. Physicians are the decision makers who determine who gains access to what services and when. Why, then, don't they control the organized systems of delivery now? Perhaps, like engineers in the aerospace industry or finance experts in banking, they find technical expertise an insufficient basis for claiming control. Still, unlike engineers or accountants, physicians are individual entrepreneurs. They work within systems and institutions as powerful insiders, though usually not as employees. While this status gives physicians considerable autonomy, it also decreases the likelihood that they will take control of the systems themselves.

For example, hospitals have attempted to replicate engineer and accountant relationships by acquiring physician practices, purchasing their assets, managing their practices, and forming various legal structures to align physicians more closely with hospital systems. The intent is to place physicians within their bureaucratic structures and to create unified provider combinations capable of competing effectively for managed care contracts. Managed care organizations have also experimented with such arrangements, though so far they appear more inclined to pursue contractual arrangements with physician networks, independent practice organizations, and group practices.

Despite such strategies, physicians usually retain their independence as professionals. We suspect that in the long run physicians will be controlled primarily by physicians. If—and only if—they consolidate into larger and larger organizations, they may begin to replace hospitals in controlling the integration of delivery in the local market.

Consolidation

Physicians are joining a number and variety of organizations, often belonging to more than one competitive entity at a time. It is not unlikely, for example, for a physician to be a member of a major group practice that is part of a national PPMC, a hospital PHO that is a member of a system-wide "super PHO," and one or more local IPAs and networks.

There are few reliable sources of information on the numbers of physician entities or on the numbers of physicians within them. Estimates range from 2,000 to 3,000 IPAs and a similar number of PHOs nationally, with over half of practicing physicians in one or more such organizational entities. An emerging model is for a major multispecialty physician group practice to take the lead in organizing IPAs. The physician practice would become the hub in a hub/spoke arrangement, while IPA members would form the spokes. In the future, physician-initiated and -controlled structures like these could easily challenge the positions of the forming hub/spoke structures of strategic hospital alliances.

In the long run, the only way for physicians to challenge strategic hospital alliances and managed care organizations is to form into more tightly structured organizations, namely, physician group practices. Looser alliances, such as PHOs, can facilitate contracting arrangements, but to gain control over the delivery structures and to facilitate access to needed capital for development, physicians will need to form their own strategic entities. These, we suggest, will likely be large physician group practices, which themselves will align with still larger IPAs.

The American Medical Association (AMA) provides a listing of group practices in its Physician Masterfile—with 46,959 entries, perhaps the most comprehensive available. After eliminating entries designated as "ineligible" (for a variety of reasons, including dissolutions, duplications, and those not meeting AMA definitions), the AMA estimates that there are 19,787 "eligible" groups in the United States. They define a physician group as

> . . . three or more physicians [providing health care services] who are formally organized as a legal entity in which business and clinical facilities, records, and personnel are shared. Income from medical services provided by the group are treated as receipts of the group and distributed according to some prearranged plan. (Havlicek 1996, p. 1)

This definition excludes several classes of groups likely to be important strategically. In particular, it excludes hospital and/or hospital system groups that directly employ physicians, as well as groups that are within group model HMOs. The definition does, however, include groups that are part of staff model HMOs.

Combining their 1994/1995 Census of Medical Groups with the Masterfile data, the AMA estimates that there are 210,811 physicians in those 19,787 physician group practices. This represents an estimated 34.4 percent of all nonfederal physicians (Havlicek 1996). The AMA also estimates that, as of 1995, the mean number of physicians per group was 10.5 (up only slightly from a mean of 9.1 per group as of 1984), while the median was 5.0. These numbers suggest that physician groups may be far behind hospital and managed care rivals in consolidating their markets.

Because a three-person group does not constitute a major threat except, perhaps, in very small communities or specific specialties, we prefer to look at groups that are large enough to affect the behaviors of other physician organizations, hospital systems, and managed care organizations. These larger groups have greater prospects for assuming leadership over the delivery networks and systems forming at the local level. To examine these, we draw upon our own unique database of "strategically important" physician group practices nationwide. We equate strategic importance with being "large," which we arbitrarily define as groups with 20 or more physicians. Although not all such groups are strategically important, at least not yet, some of the larger ones are very powerful players, particularly in such markets as Los Angeles and Minneapolis (Penner 1997).

Focusing on the urban areas, where over 80 percent of all practicing physicians are located, we estimate that there are just over 1,700 large (20 or more physicians) groups. These groups include nearly 160,000 physicians, or 32 percent of the approximately 500,000 physicians working in urban areas. Table 2.6 summarizes the percentages of physicians in these large groups by market size and region.

Interestingly, these patterns differ from those for managed care and hospital SHA penetration in the urban markets. While there is some positive association with market size, the differences across market size categories are minimal. Variations across region are much greater, with about 40 percent of urban physicians in the Midwest and West being in large groups. The south and especially the Northeast fall far short of these levels, despite the presence of many large academic-based groups in the Northeast.

An important trend in physician group formation is the emergence of PPMCs, adding a new dimension to the consolidation of physician markets (Burns et al. 1997). By combining many physician practices, single and group, into larger companies, *PPMCs offer potentially the greatest single force for restructuring physician markets and reallocating power at the local market level.* To date, PPMCs have had minimal impact on concentration locally, with the possible exception of Southern California. Their potential for growth, however, is great, given their ability to acquire capital from individual investors and through issuance of stock. Indeed, mergers like the one recently discussed (but never com-

TABLE 2.6. Large physician group practice penetration in Metropolitan Statistical Areas (percentage of MSA physicians by market size and region).

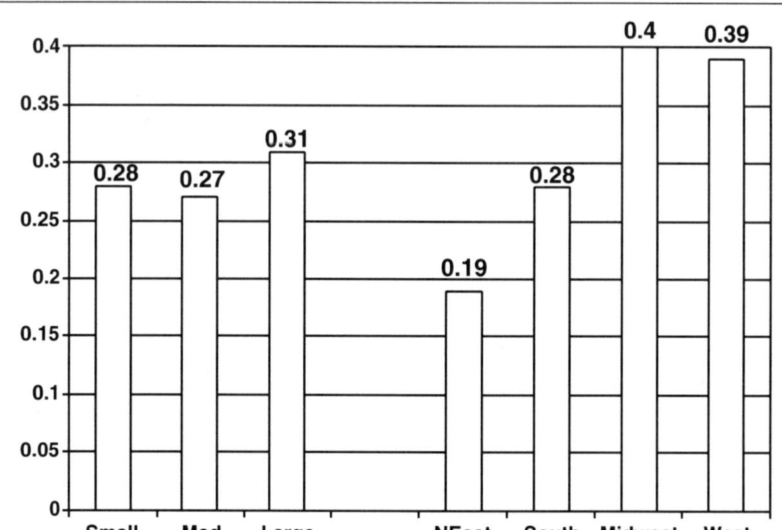

pleted) by the nation's two largest PPMCs, MedPartners and Phycor, could create powerful new players and catalyze further consolidation in physician markets. To the extent this occurs, tensions between physician groups and hospital systems could erupt into full-fledged warfare and force the question of who will broker managed care contracts and control the systems for integrating health care.

Although it is common to focus on the small number of PPMCs that have gone public, the number is fairly large if all multipractice groups are included in the count. Given that hospital-based groups characteristically contain a number of individual practices, it is quite possible that most large practices already have multiple practice sites as well as expansion potential. Clearly, we must follow these groups over time to assess trends in physician group formation and market consolidation.

Entry Barriers

As is the case in other sectors, judgments regarding entry barriers are subjective. Physicians coming out of school face licensure, certification, and other barriers to practice. Physicians moving into a new area must be concerned about establishing referral relationships, acquiring hospital privileges, and attracting patients. Although physician oversupply may impact entry (Begun and Luke 1997) in some specialties and certain oversupplied markets, there are few entry barriers in general. Since most markets are still somewhat fragmented, opportunities exist for new organizations (e.g., PPMCs and hospital-based management companies) to assist groups in forming or acquiring practices. The barrier for them is mostly the current high level of fragmentation that exists in most physician markets. It is one thing to acquire a large, thriving group and quite another to convince large numbers of physicians practicing in solo or small group practices to join a PPMC. For this reason, it is likely that PPMCs will seek out the existing large groups to consolidate markets in the future (as MedPartners did in the Southern California area).

Product Differentiation

Overall, there is a high level of product differentiation within physician markets. Physicians enjoy unique locations, selective hospital privileges, distinctive specialties, and informal and often highly personal relationships with their patients. In addition, many physicians are associated with distinctive networks, groups, IPAs, PHOs, and many other physician organizations. All these factors give physicians added leverage within their markets.

Summary

Because of its fragmented structure, high product differentiation, and low entry barriers, the physician sector is best considered monopolistically competitive. Such markets generally have a large number of competitors who enjoy high levels of distinctiveness, giving them considerable market power individually despite the large numbers.

Given continued growth in this sector and the rise of large physician groups and practice management companies, physicians appear to be headed toward an oligopoly structure (small numbers of highly interdependent competitors). How long it will take to get there is unknown, and this sector could remain highly fragmented for the foreseeable future. The degree to which physicians consolidate could be the single most important strategic question remaining in health care. We believe that what happens in the physician sector will do much to determine the ultimate structures of all healthcare markets well into the next century.

Market Stages—Going Beyond Horizontal

In 1993, in those long-ago beginnings of market restructuring in health care, the University HealthSystem Consortium contracted with APM, a consulting firm, to study the changing healthcare markets and derive implications for the nation's academic teaching hospitals. During the study, APM proposed that the markets are moving through distinct stages on their way to some idealized last stage of managed competition (APM 1995). The stages concept has been redone by others (Coile 1997; Voluntary Hospitals of America 1994), but the essential feature of all such models is a sequence of steps leading to a final, highly structured stage of market restructuring. Although APM did not present an in-depth analysis of the stages' logic, others are currently examining this matter more systematically (see Burns et al. 1997). To conclude this chapter and acknowledge the currency of the stages model, we offer a few relevant observations.

In his presentation of five market stages, Coile suggested that managed care penetration is the trigger that moves markets from one stage to the next. His stages and trigger points are shown in Table 2.7.

We set aside the question of how Coile arrived at the trigger points to raise a more basic question: What is the likelihood that markets will move in some systematic fashion across a predetermined series of stages as levels of managed care penetration increase? Because managed care includes a wide range of payment mechanisms and arrangements between payers and providers, we have no basis for concluding that payment will necessarily shift toward capitation or that group and/or staff model HMOs will flourish.

What do we know about the association between managed care penetration and system and market restructuring? In Table 2.8, we provide the correlation coefficients that indicate the degree to which hospital-based SHAs and physician participation in large groups are associated with the variance across markets in the level of managed care penetration (for a more extensive analysis, see Burns et al. 1997).

As the table shows, the correlation coefficients are fairly small, ranging between .09 and .15. The correlations between each of these and the log of the MSA population, however, are nearly four times the size of the direct correlations between the three market structural indicators (except for the correlation with large physician group penetration, which is relatively unassociated with market size).

What does this tell us? First, provider restructuring is only slightly associated with managed care penetration. Second, market size may be a far stronger predictor of market restructuring than the so-called stages construct. Larger markets experience much more HMO penetration, SHA formation, and, to a somewhat lesser extent, large physician group formation than do smaller markets.

There is certainly the possibility, as predicted by the stages model, that provider horizontal strategies will eventually give way to vertically structured, comprehensive delivery systems. If these systems were then to begin contracting directly with the ultimate buyers—eliminating the middleman and the insurers—this would be fully consistent with both the stages models and the 1990s paradigm shift hypothesis. Enthusiastic about the possibility of systems forming in this way, Coile said:

> Provider-sponsored networks (PSNs) could be every hospital administrator's and physician's dream: contracting for patients directly with employers and government without an intermediary, HMO, insurance plan, or third-party administrator. . . . The PSN movement is providers' direct counterattack against managed care plans, after years of discounting and controls. . . . (1997, pp. 83, 85)

TABLE 2.7. Stages of HMO penetration.

Stage	HMO penetration
Stage 1: Can't Spell HMO	Less than 5%
Stage 2: Managed Care Gets Aggressive	5–14%
Stage 3: Managed Care Penetration	15–24%
Stage 4: Managed Competition	25–40%
Stage 5: Post-Reform	Greater than 40%

Source: Coile 1997.

TABLE 2.8. Correlations among structural indicators—Evidence for stages model?

	HMO Penn	SHA Penn	Lg Phy Gp Penn
HMO Penn	—	—	—
SHA Penn	.16	—	—
Lg Phy Gp Penn	.21	.16	—
Log MSA Pop	.47	.46	.18

We believe vertical system formation and direct contracting would be more than a "counterattack"; rather, *they would dramatically restructure the industry, with consequences not yet fully envisioned.* There are strong signals that this could happen. Consider the business coalition in Minneapolis that announced plans to enter into direct contracting with provider and insurer-based healthcare networks. Note legislative discussions at the federal level that could open the door to direct contracting on the part of providers. Also, as we discussed in this chapter, there are perhaps more indicators that the full vertical structuring will be slow at best.

Even if further vertical and horizontal structuring come to pass, one key question remains: Which players will ultimately form and control the forming systems? We foresee battles where one of the three main healthcare players—insurers, hospital systems, and physician groups—take actions that undermine the ability of their rivals to form and market competitive networks. Whatever the case, it is within such scenarios that the stages models have the greatest promise. Today, however, the healthcare markets are very distant indeed from the last stage predicted for market restructuring—a stage we hold at this point to be almost mythical in proportion and significance.

References

APM/University HealthSystem Consortium. 1995. "How Markets Evolve." *Hospitals & Health Networks* 69(5), March 5.

Begun, J.W. and R.D. Luke. 1997. "Physician Right Sizing: Origins, Processes and Consequences." Paper commissioned by the Center for Health Management Research, Industry Advisory Board (under review).

Burns, R.B., G.J. Bazzoli, L. Dynan, and D.R. Wholey. 1997. "Managed Care Market Stages, and Integrated Systems: Is There a Relationship?" *Health Affairs* 16(6), November/December: 204–218.

Burns, R.B. and J.C. Robinson. 1997. "Physician Practice Management Companies: Implications for Hospital-Based Integrated Delivery Systems." *Frontiers of Health Services Management,* Winter: 3–35.

Christianson, J.B., R.D. Feldman, and D.R. Wholey. 1997. "HMO Mergers: Estimating Impacts on Premiums and Costs." *Health Affairs* 16(6), November/December: 133–141.

Coile, R.C., Jr. 1997. *The Five Stages of Managed Care: Strategies for Providers, HMOs, and Suppliers.* Chicago: Health Administration Press.

CSC Consulting. 1996. *Efficient Healthcare Consumer Response: Improving the Efficiency of the Healthcare Supply Chain.* Waltham, Mass.: CSC, November.

Gabel, J. 1997. "Ten Ways HMOs Have Changed During the 1990s." *Health Affairs,* May/June: 134–145.

Havlicek, P.L. 1996. *Medical Groups in the U.S.: A Survey of Practice Characteristics, 1996 Edition.* Chicago: American Medical Association.

InterStudy. (1997). *The InterStudy Competitive Edge, 4.* Minneapolis, Minn.: InterStudy.

Lamphere, J.A., P. Neuman, K. Langwell, and D. Sherman. 1997. "The Surge in Medicare Managed Care, An Update." *Health Affairs,* May/June: 127–133.

Penner, M.J. 1997. *Capitation in California: A Study of Physician Organizations Managing Risk.* Chicago: Health Administration Press.

Porter, M.E. 1980. *Competitive Strategy: Techniques for Analyzing Industries and Competitors.* New York: Free Press.

Robinson, J.C. and L.P. Casalino. 1995. "The Growth of Medical Groups Paid Through Capitation in California." *New England Journal of Medicine* 333(25), December 21, 1684–87.

Voluntary Hospitals of America. 1994. *Integration: Market Forces and Critical Success Factors.* Dallas: VHA.

Williamson Institute. 1997. Database on health systems and markets. http://www.vcu.edu/haeweb/wi/websites.html

3

Strategy Analyses and Implications for Information Systems

ROICE D. LUKE AND RAMESH K. SHUKLA

With the healthcare markets in the midst of major changes, it is difficult to predict exactly what strategies will ensure competitive advantage in the long run. Despite this uncertainty, individual organizations must find ways to compete effectively. However, what strategies they should pursue will depend on evaluations of their own and their competitors' strengths and weaknesses, as well as careful assessments of their market environments.

If questions about organizational form and strategy are difficult to answer in a rapidly changing environment, what can be said about information system strategies? It is reasonable to assume that investments in information systems will depend directly on the outcomes of organizational change and strategic decision making. To the extent this is true, the critical decisions on information systems may need to be deferred until the broader strategies are resolved. It is possible, of course, that cause and effect will be reversed. Information systems could play a more catalytic role, facilitating organizational restructuring, opening up ways by which integration might be made to work, and providing a means for achieving competitive advantage.

In this chapter, we move from a broad to a narrow treatment of healthcare strategy and markets. Our primary purpose is to provide the concepts and frameworks needed for healthcare executives to assess strategy for their own organizations and within their own markets. We also examine in this chapter how some critical trends in the markets, as described in Chapter 2, apply to the analysis of strategy. At the end of the chapter, we explore the relationships between the broader strategies of organizations and their investments in information systems.

Analytic Framework: The Positioning School

As a framework for this chapter, we adopt what Mintzberg labeled the "positioning" school of strategy formulation. This perspective, he suggests, is one of three major schools, the others being the "design" and "planning" schools. Unlike the latter two, the positioning school "focuses on the content of the strategies (differentiation, diversification, etc.) more than on the processes by which they are prescribed to be made (which are generally assumed, often implicitly, to be those of the planning school)" (Mintzberg 1994, p. 3). The positioning school thus directs attention to strategy itself and, importantly, to the analytic relationships between strategy and market structure. As a result, this perspective, relative to the other two, is best suited for formulating strategy under conditions of environmental uncertainty (Mintzberg 1990), such as exists in the healthcare field today.

Mintzberg notes that the planning school is limited, primarily because of a tendency toward inflexibility and excessive reliance on projections based on data from the recent past. By contrast, the special quality of the positioning school is that it directs attention to the markets and the interplay among rivals and other players within the markets. Under conditions of uncertainty, an accurate though possibly not fully corroborated view of reality will generally be preferred to a precise firing at a wrong target.

Figure 3.1 presents the industrial organization framework on which the positioning school is founded. The key relationship, between market structure and the conduct of firms, is equated with the making of strategy. Market structure and the conduct of firms, both drivers of performance, are affected by environmental factors and have played significant roles in the healthcare field in the 1990s. An important feedback effect identified in the figure is the impact of conduct or strategy on market structure itself. This reverse relationship is perhaps best illustrated by both the hospital and managed care sectors, where mergers, acquisitions, and other combinations (conduct/strategy) have increased the concentration in the markets (structure). In response, physicians have joined with groups and/or practice management companies and aligned with other players at the local market level, thus increasing the levels of concentration in their markets as well.

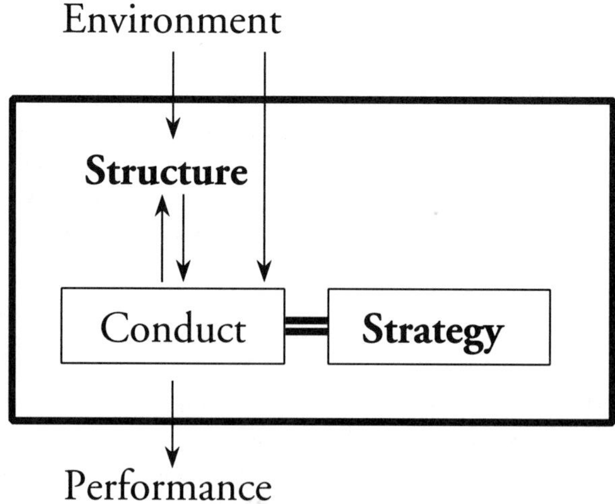

FIGURE 3.1. Industrial Organization Paradigm: A Framework for Strategy Analysis

Strategic Visions in Health Care

For long-term success, any organization needs strategic visions, no matter how they are generated. In times of high uncertainty, few organizations can survive without a well-reasoned sense of direction. Strategic visions are the conceptual representation of the overarching relationships between strategy and market structure.

Commenting on strategic visions, Mintzberg observed:

> . . . if you have no vision but only formal plans, then every unpredicted change in the environment makes you feel like your sky is falling. It comes as a fitting lesson, therefore, that the Japanese have been able to impose so much of that "turbulence" on American business in good part because they have been informal learners more than formal strategic planners. (1994, p. 210)

An organization's strategy may be complicated and groundbreaking, or it may be as simple as holding the course or improving what has worked well in the recent past. "Pizzazz" is not a prerequisite for a valid vision, as was recognized by Charles Wang, one of the founders of Computer Associates. How did his software company come to reap over $3 billion in annual sales? The company's vision was key, he suggested, but that vision was not particularly elaborate:

> People ask us, "In the beginning, what was your vision?" Our vision? Meet payroll next week. That was our big vision. We took it a week at a time. And you do whatever is necessary. (quoted in Jager and Ortiz 1997, p. 129)

It is not uncommon, of course, for strategic perspectives to be crowned as visionary in retrospect, especially if they prove to be successful. No matter how "ordinary" they may seem, they deserve that crown every bit as much as do ground-breaking innovations that blast an organization "out of the box." It is true that ordinary visions may lack the kind of star quality that generates excitement and produces radical departures from existing organizational strategies. *The goal of visions, however, is not to excite, but to identify those things organizations need to do to survive and thrive in their markets.* Uninteresting visions are not necessarily less valuable.

Still, strategic visions that are focused exclusively on approaches to achieving competitive advantage may not produce the anticipated levels of performance, organizational unity, or commitment. For most organizations, strategic visions should go beyond mere insights into strategy; they also must embody an organization's overall values and missions. In his book on strategic vision, Quigley wrote:

> The corporate vision is the most fundamental statement of a corporation's values, aspirations, and goals. It is an appeal to its members' hearts and minds. It must indicate a clear understanding of where the corporation is today and offer a road map for the future. (1993, pp. 5–6)

In this sense, strategic visions are tied inextricably to an organization's culture. While Quigley recognized that no organization can survive for long without an appropriate business strategy, he also stressed the need to join that strategy to the hearts and minds of an organization's members. Strategic visions, therefore, can inspire and unify organizations if they are transformed into expectations, molded into strong corporate cultures, and grounded in shared and positive values and purposes.

Defining the Vision

Many executives wrestle endlessly with the concept of "vision." Some experience moments when the clouds part and grand strategies form in their minds. Others discover their visions only at the end of extended analytic investigations, their visions emerging not as brilliant insights, but as conclusions, summations, or endpoints to the analysis of strategy. For still others, strategic visions appear never to emerge. While these executives may have failed to conceptualize and analyze their market environments, it is possible that their ideal strategies were dismissed because they lacked the excitement associated with "real" strategic visions.

As many executives have already discovered, visioning the future and deriving implications for strategy is not an easy process. Accordingly, the leaders of organizations need to build routines into their work experiences in which they regularly reflect on market dynamics and assumptions underlying their chosen strategies. These activities should be supplemented by timely monitoring of the best thinking in the field, but with an eye to adapting what they learn to the uniqueness of their own market environments. It is simply too often the case that busy executives grab the hottest idea circulating in the field, only to find that it either does not apply to their situation or is based on popular but untested conclusions drawn from short-term industry trends.

We argue that visioning is not so much a pure creative act as it is an intellectual accomplishment firmly grounded in a definitive understanding of the interrelationships between strategy, market structure, and the distinctive capabilities of one's own organization and of one's rivals. Strategic visions, then, are all-encompassing in the sense that they embrace and extend an organization's strategies. They are usually conceptual and, for the most part, very simple. They both build and draw upon an organization's culture and structure of values. But mostly, they are derived from careful analyses of internal and external environments.

The Downside of Visions

Shared perceptions about where the markets are going and what organizations should do in response can produce some very powerful pressures for acceptance and conformity. This is the downside of visions, whether they are articulated at industry or corporate levels. Too often, visions assume an almost sacred aura, becoming nearly untouchable. Sometimes this happens because industry spokespersons or influentials give them credence or, at the corporate level, because they are advocated by charismatic leaders whose views of the future are accepted with little challenge and pursued despite growing evidence to the contrary.

The risk of industry visions "catching on," regardless of their validity, is greatest in environments that are rapidly changing and uncertain. These volatile market environments recently have been conceptualized under the term *hypercompetition* (D'Aveni 1994). A central proposition of hypercompetition is that *strategies must be continually reconsidered and revised, since few competitive advantages can be sustained for long.* Unfortunately, in the rush to find new sources of advantage, competitors will often duplicate the approaches of others without discerning whether or not the duplicated strategies fit their own organizational needs. This point was underscored by Michael Porter:

> Unnerved by forecasts of hypercompetition, managers increase its likelihood by imitating everything about their competitors. Exhorted to think in terms of revolution, managers chase every new technology for its own sake. . . . Companies imitate one another in a type of herd behavior, each assuming rivals know something they do not. (Porter 1996, p. 75)

To some extent, this herd mentality is a function of taking insufficient time to conduct one's own assessments. Collective wisdom often fails to recognize this as one of the many underlying factors that, in the end, militate against the full realization of accepted visions.

Lessons from the Computer Industry: The Java Effect

Before we continue discussing strategy formulation for healthcare organizations, let us take a brief look at desktop computing, another industry in which assumptions about strategy must be reevaluated constantly. Analysis of the strategic issues facing competitors in this industry should provide some important insights into our own industry.

Desktop computing resembles health care in several ways. Integration and the control of the integrative processes are strategic imperatives in this industry as much as they are in health care, if not more. In both industries, the strategic power of integration also could be undermined as new and unexpected developments weaken the currently accepted rationale for coordination and control.

Microsoft versus Java

At the center of the integration question in desktop computing is the concept of the "platform." Control of platforms can be critical in this industry, since the platforms shape the development of applications and govern the linkages among computers and accessories. It is akin to controlling the center of the board in chess—by dominating the center, one forces all opponents to the periphery, where strategic moves are constrained and marginalized.

Microsoft currently rules desktop publishing, primarily because it defeated rivals in the platform battle and thereby emerged as the "standard" (Wallace 1997; Gates 1995; Cringely 1996). Microsoft's growing position in the market, however, is by no means unassailable. An ominous threat looms on the horizon: Java, a new "platform-independent" software developed by Microsoft's arch rival, Sun. The threat of Java is not that it would produce an alternative operating system, but that it would offer a substitute mechanism by which the power of integration could be neutralized. With this universal language, one could acquire any operating system and still have access to the breadth of applications available in the industry—a revolutionary concept that could reduce Microsoft's operating systems to mere commodities. Add to this the threat of Internet distribution mechanisms like Netscape, the leading provider of Internet browsers, and one can see how Microsoft could be forced to compete on the basis of price and quality, its monopolistic position being eroded by Java and the Internet.

The Java Effect in Health Care

Is there a "Java" lurking in the healthcare industry? What has the power to untie the local linkages of vertical and horizontal integration, fragmenting the system and network monoliths and transforming their individual components to commodity status? Consider first the local hospital systems. Since the early 1990s, they have aggressively attempted to become the "platforms" of health care by controlling the forming integrated systems. If one were to view the hospital companies as analogous to IBM, the dominating hardware "box maker" of the 1980s, one could visualize the possibility of an "operating system" (analogous to Microsoft with its DOS and Windows products) emerging that could dislodge them as the controlling platforms for integrating delivery at the local market level.

Perhaps more important, though, is this question: Is there a Java equivalent that could make integration, whether controlled by hospitals, physicians, or insurance organizations, superfluous and costly? So far, the insurance companies have been able to pick and choose among many of the providers assembled within so-called integrated delivery systems, thus neutralizing their ability to act as single entities or to translate integration into tangible competitive advantages. Of course, this capability could disappear altogether once the integrated systems become fully formed and systems for internal control are implemented. At the present time, however, the insurers' demonstrated ability to contract with individual system members seriously erodes the market positions of integrated systems, fragments their vertical structures, and, consequently, converts their individual components to commodity status—the Java effect!

There is also the possibility that sufficient integration could be achieved by the mere formation of networks and other loosely structured grouping mechanisms and the linking of all members within them via standardized information systems. In other words, we may find that the goals of integration can be achieved without the costly imposition of heavily layered hierarchical structures (as might be needed for the fully integrated systems to work)—a possible second Java effect.

Finally, there are clear indications of cracks at the surface of the integrated delivery system paradigm itself. InterStudy, the managed care data company, early on reported that the much-heralded staff model and group model health maintenance organizations (HMOs) were declining in their share of the HMO market and that the more loosely structured HMOs—independent practice associations (IPAs), point-of-service plans (POSs), mixed models, and network models—were emerging as the favored choices of consumers (InterStudy 1994). Add to this the specific case of the prototype integrated system, Kaiser Permanente, which has moved gradually from an ideological commitment to the integration of health plans, physicians, and hospitals to a strategy where neither ownership of hospitals nor tight relationships with all participating physicians is considered essential. Their recent development of POS products and the countermoves by their physicians to organize an independent national organization—the Permanente Federation—speaks volumes about the limitations of the idealized integrated model.

Seamless, powerful integrated delivery systems are difficult to develop and maintain, but there have been some notable success stories. These include both tight and loose organizational models and range across markets nationwide. Systems like Intermountain Healthcare in Salt Lake City, Sentara in Norfolk, Promina in Atlanta, Henry Ford in Detroit, and Community Health Systems in Houston have transformed the vision of the accepted paradigm into credible competitive advantages.

In sum, the paradigm of the 1990s is clouded and changing. The challenge facing healthcare strategists, therefore, is to extract and build upon those parts of the vision that fit their organizations and the realities of their markets. We all would be well advised to keep our collective eyes on the core concepts and interrelationships of the accepted paradigm to see if the platforms of integration sustain the promised advantages and remain in the future the strategies of choice at the local market level.

Strategy in a Competitive Market

In a perfect world, one might hope that industry restructuring would follow a grand design, driven by the trinity of social rationality—efficiency, quality, and access. In a competitive world, however, strategy is more likely to be the driver of market restructuring.

We define strategy as *"those concepts and ideas that guide an organization in its attempts to achieve competitive advantage over rivals."* The "competitive" part centers strategy directly within a market environment, and the "advantage" part draws attention to the ways in which organizations distinguish themselves to compete within their markets. This particular definition assumes an oligopolistic market structure, which characterizes the structures of managed care, hospital markets, and, possibly over time, physician markets. Because of small numbers, the competitors (the oligopolists) tend to be highly interdependent with and reactive to the strategic moves of one another. For this reason, the phrase "over rivals" is included in the definition of strategy.

Gaining Competitive Advantage

The literature is full of approaches to achieving competitive advantage, ranging from marketing tactics to internal restructuring and reengineering. Porter (1996) identified two primary camps that accent different approaches to achieving competitive advantage: those emphasizing building competitive positions within markets (his preferred perspective), and those embracing the need to improve internal capabilities and performance as a primary competitive strategy. The latter gained considerable ascendancy in the 1980s, largely as a reflexive reaction to the successes of Japanese firms in the emerging global economy. Healthcare organizations have not been immune to this movement.

While it is useful to distinguish between internal and external sources of competitive advantage, it is less helpful to view them as in opposition to one another. *One can strengthen the other, and both may be necessary for success.* The importance of both internal and external sources of competitive advantage is reflected in that well-known strategy acronym, SWOT, where *s*trengths and *w*eaknesses take on an internal focus and *o*pportunities and *t*hreats, an external focus. All are essential to achieving competitive advantage, especially in turbulent market environments.

The Five "Ps"

There are at least five sources of competitive advantage, which we call the five "Ps":

- **Power**—gained through the accumulation and effective consolidation of mass
- **Position**—gained by achieving distinctive value in the minds of consumers
- **Pace**—gained through managing the timing and intensity of actions
- **Potential**—derived from the accumulation of critical resources and capabilities
- **Performance**—gained through the efficient conduct of operations and the effective implementation of strategy.

As Figure 3.2 shows, power and position are primarily external sources of advantage, while potential and performance are primarily internal. Pace applies equally to both levels.

Power

Power strategies are among the most commonly discussed in the literature and frequently pursued in practice. Because they build on the advantages of sheer mass (market power, economies of scale, etc.), power strategies are fundamental to oligopoly competition. The strategy of building mass is especially important for firms competing in markets that are consolidating, as is the case for most healthcare markets.

By contrast, in monopolistically competitive markets (markets with many competitors, each of which enjoys some degree of product differentiation and, there-

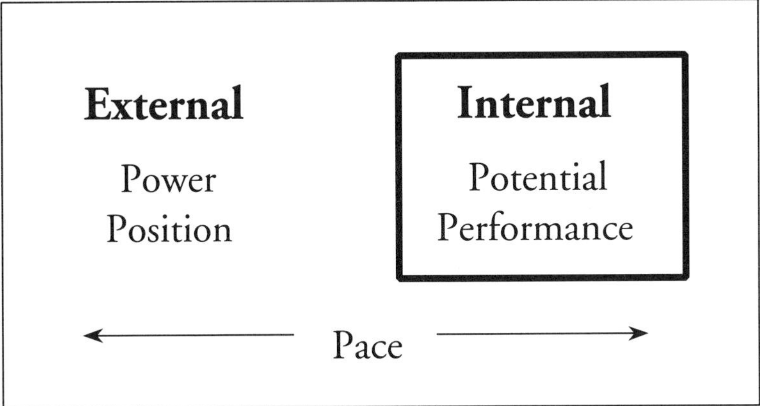

FIGURE 3.2. Strategy: Identifying Sources of Competitive Advantage

fore, market power), power per se may take a somewhat lower priority. Because they are relatively small and protected by distinctive product characteristics (location, specialty, quality, etc.), competitors within such markets tend to be more focused on winning consumers than defeating rivals. However, if rivals in monopolistically competitive markets see ways by which consolidation might gain immediate advantages, power strategies could become of preeminent importance (which appears may be the case in the physician sector).

Four strategies are of particular importance in the power strategy category:

- **Horizontal expansion**—expansion in the scale of existing business activities (e.g., merger of two hospitals)
- **Horizontal integration**—the pursuit of synergies among different types of businesses that are not vertically related (e.g., jointly managing nursing home and hospital businesses)
- **Vertical integration**—the pursuit of synergies among different types of businesses that share input-output relationships (e.g., integrating hospital and managed care businesses)
- **Portfolio**—the pursuit of financial synergies among different types of businesses (e.g., combining any businesses primarily for financial purposes).

Most of these have been prominent in the restructuring healthcare markets of the 1990s, as competitors have sought to reap advantages by building complex and often dominating healthcare systems.

The importance of local markets to healthcare competition suggests the need to distinguish between *relative* and *absolute* power. A strategy that leads to the building of large-scale organizations—for example, national strategies pursued by Columbia/HCA or a merger between Phycor and MedPartners (which has since been called off)—derives its rationale from the advantages of absolute power. On the other hand, one that amasses local market shares without regard to organizational scale—for example, most of the local hospital systems that have formed across the country—derives advantages from power *relative* to the competitors in a given market. Hospital and physician competitors have actively pursued relative power in recent years, while managed care firms have tended to combine absolute with relative power strategies. Nonprofit hospitals have placed particular emphasis on the advantages of local market dominance (relative power). With this source of advantage, they have competed quite successfully against the small number of nationally expanded hospital firms.

The advantages of absolute power have yet to be demonstrated within the provider sector, but the increasing strength of the physician practice management companies (PPMCs) could yet establish the advantages of absolute power among physicians. Through their participation in PPMCs, local physician practices appear to gain much-needed managerial capabilities as well as access to capital, information systems, and other infrastructure support. As they grow, the PPMCs will also gain advantages in negotiating for contracts and, possibly, in controlling the integrative "platforms" of local health care.

Position

According to Porter, one reason the Japanese competitive threat is now running out of steam is the fact that they have paid too little attention to positioning, having assumed that their advantages in operational efficiencies could not be duplicated (1996, p. 63) or overcome. As firms worldwide have improved their production processes, Japanese firms, he suggests, have been unable to distinguish themselves from their rivals in the increasingly globalized economy.

The primary options within position strategy include distinguishing an organization or its products by:

- offering low cost
- achieving high differentiation
- serving unique customer niches.

Over the years, competitors in health care have tended to compete on the basis of the last two options, having generally eschewed low-cost positions. Consumer fears have played a large role in this omission. Despite the fact that low cost could be equated with managerial effectiveness, there is growing evidence that consumers still associate strong low-cost positioning with quality-diminishing restrictions on utilization. HMOs have experienced particular difficulties in effectively projecting low cost position, as consumers have reacted by interpreting these as efforts to constrain utilization, avoid coverage, limit access, or lower the overall quality of care

Ironically, despite the obvious importance of quality for healthcare providers, few have been able to establish distinctive quality positions either. The academic medical centers located in many large northeastern markets may be an exception, but because many of these also serve as the healthcare "safety nets" for the poor and disadvantaged, they have difficulty capitalizing on their ready-made positions of high quality. The expansion of the Minnesota-based Mayo Clinic into Arizona and Florida clearly appears to be based on a strategy grounded on quality positioning. It will be interesting to see if they succeed in this and if others will follow their lead by seeking to establish strong quality positions in their markets.

The forming integrated systems also are attempting to extend advantages gained from their growing size and complexity to capture high quality positions within their markets. In time, this may work for them, especially if they can market their enlarged local profiles effectively and use improvements gained from their management reforms to enhance their reputations for quality. If, in addition, they are successful in capturing the limited number of top-quality clinicians and institutions available in most markets, this strategy could prove hard to beat. On the other hand, these strategies could remain rather transparent, as patients retain a focus on individual caregivers and institutions.

Pace

Timing—our pace strategy—has long been recognized as a critical dimension of strategy, encompassing such concepts as surprise, signaling, and momentum (Amburgey and Miner 1989; Harrigan 1985). Early movers can gain considerable advantage, assuming they have assessed the environment properly. The danger, of course, is in misreading the economics of restructuring and making moves that prove costly and produce few tangible competitive advantages.

Miles and Snow (1978) constructed one of the most interesting typologies of pace strategies nearly 20 years ago. They classified organizations according to the degree to which they were willing to assume risk or to take aggressive action in pursuing strategy. They identified four different types:

- **Prospectors**—organizations that frequently search for new market opportunities and regularly engage in experimentation and innovation
- **Analyzers**—organizations that maintain stable operations in some areas but also search for new opportunities, often following the lead of prospector organizations
- **Defenders**—organizations that search for additional opportunities for growth and seldom make adjustments to existing, well-established strategies
- **Reactors**—organizations that perceive opportunities and turbulence, but are not able to adapt consistently or effectively.

The evidence is mixed as to the relative success of these strategic orientations. Several "leading" healthcare organizations (Phycor of Nashville, Intermountain Healthcare in Salt Lake City, and Sentara in Norfolk) appear to have gained considerable advantage by becoming first movers. There are, however, a number of high-profile examples of organizations that have not been successful as prospectors: Humana, with its entry into managed care in the 1980s; Columbia/HCA in its attempt to acquire Blue Cross of Ohio; and Coastal, with its difficulties in combining physician and managed care businesses in Florida.

In the end, an organization's visionary leaders will be the ones most challenged by the strategies of pace. They will need to determine not only what their organizations require to gain competitive advantage, but also when actions should be taken. There is obvious comfort in remaining cautious; however, there is also satisfaction in taking bold actions, especially when they achieve their intended effects. In turbulent environments, on the other hand, pace strategies could be among the most important of the five major sources of competitive advantage. The relics of both early and late movers strew the landscapes of hypercompetitive environments.

Potential

Potential refers to the distinctive resources and capabilities that might give an organization an advantage as it designs and implements its strategies. Some organizations enjoy unique locations or distinctive strengths in certain specialty areas. Others gain from their memberships in multihospital systems, memberships in purchasing alliances, advanced information systems, recognized research capabilities, unique clinical resources, modern and attractive physical facilities, and/or aggressive and effective managerial talent.

Not all distinctive capabilities, however, can be transformed into competitive advantages. Collis and Montgomery (1995) identified some essential characteristics that may be needed for a resource or capability to become important strategically:

- **Transferability**—it can be transformed into a resource or service that is valued by customers (correlation with positioning)
- **Competitive superiority**—it is truly better than the resources or capabilities of competitors
- **Inimitability**—it cannot be copied easily by competitors
- **Substitutability**—it cannot be trumped through substitution by competitors
- **Durability**—its value does not depreciate quickly.

The resources or capabilities of many competitors may not pass such market tests, or they simply may be unable to sustain competitive advantages. Nevertheless, like quality positioning, this is an area that may be inadequately mined by healthcare strategists. Many healthcare providers have tangible and intangible assets that go largely undeveloped from a strategic perspective. *In fact, viable external strategies may emerge only after organizations fully exploit their internal strengths and shore up their weaknesses.* Too often, organizations go through the motions of assessing their strengths and weaknesses without acting sufficiently on their conclusions. External strategies often have a greater appeal.

Performance

Closely associated with potential as a source of advantage is the effectiveness with which strategies are implemented and organizations are managed. Implementation and operations are often the keys to successful strategies. Many great ideas have fallen far short of potential because they failed to ensure proper implementation.

Drawing attention to the importance of effective implementation of strategy, Porter (1996) introduced the concept of value chains. An organization's value chain is a diagrammatic disaggregation of the activities it undertakes to produce its products and services and carry out its strategies. By assessing their value chains, organizations can identify those areas where improvements in performance could lead to more successful execution of strategy.

Many organizations have invested much effort in the analysis of overall organizational processes by implementing continuous quality improvement, reengineering, and other such evaluative and improvement techniques. Similar processes, however, are rarely implemented to guide and evaluate the execution of strategies, despite the importance of strategy to organizational survival.

The need to manage and assess the implementation of strategy is especially important for integrated systems. They need to ensure not only that each individual component runs efficiently and effectively, but that each reinforces the others and supports the overall strategic goals of the organization.

Fitting the individual parts to the whole is what Porter referred to as ensuring "organizational fit" within complex organizations (1996). He argued:

> It is harder for a rival to match an array of interlocked activities than it is merely to imitate a particular sales-force approach, match a process technology, or replicate a set of product features. Positions built on systems of activities are far more sustainable than those built on individual activities. (p. 73)

This is the central objective of the integrated system—to generate advantages from the sum of individual parts. Success may rest as much on implementation as on establishing appropriate organizational structures, incentive systems, or managerial and production control systems.

Strategy and Information Systems

Finally, we turn to information systems as tools for helping healthcare organizations achieve their overall strategies. Information systems can be viewed as resources organizations use to achieve internal integration as well as external adaptation. They can be used to improve efficiency, productivity, quality of care, and internal processes focused on revenues or costs; reduce lengths of stay and turnaround times for services; enhance capabilities for capturing future markets; and monitor rivals.

At this turbulent time in the healthcare industry, it is essential that information system strategies take full consideration of the existing market environments and overall strategies of organizations. To illustrate how this might be done, we break the analysis of markets and strategy into three key factors: stability of the market, service diversification, and market diversification. Table 3.1 provides a

TABLE 3.1. Framework for analysis of information systems strategies.

Business strategies		Stability of market structures	
Service diversification	Market diversification	Stable structure	Dynamic structure
Horizontally Integrated Systems (e.g., multiple acute care facilities)	Single Market	Several hospitals in one market with little merger, acquisition, partnership, and alliance formation activity	Several hospitals in one market with aggressive merger and acquisition activity
	Multiple Markets	Several hospitals in more than one market with little merger, acquisition, partnership, and alliance formation activity	Several hospitals in more than one market with aggressive merger and acquisition activity
Vertically Integrated Systems (multiple facilities along continuum of care, e.g., diagnostic centers, clinics, acute care, home health care, nursing homes)	Single Market	Vertically integrated services in one market with little merger, acquisition, partnership, and alliance formation activity	Vertically integrated services in one market with aggressive merger and acquisition activity
	Multiple Markets	Vertically integrated services in more than one market with little merger, acquisition, partnership, and alliance formation activity	Vertically integrated services in more than one market with aggressive merger and acquisition activity

framework for formulating how information systems might be used to support both internal operations and the pursuit of external market strategies.

The *stability* of the market dimension reflects the degree of uncertainty that surrounds markets and their structures. Dynamic markets are those with considerable room for restructuring—hospitals yet to merge or form into alliances, physician markets still fragmented, and much room for entry on the managed care side. In stable markets, there is little likelihood that mergers, acquisitions, or other such activities will produce new or radically altered organizations within the markets. The markets may still experience significant competition, but the essential market and organizational structures will have been formed.

The *service diversification* dimension captures a healthcare organization's approach to system building. In the context of the rapid consolidation taking place in the healthcare industry, we identify two of the power strategies that were described earlier: horizontal integration and vertical integration. Using a horizontal expansion strategy, a hospital system may have multiple acute care facilities in a single market or in several geographically dispersed markets. A vertically integrated strategy might lead to a system in which acute care, diagnostic, ambulatory, outpatient surgery, home health, and long-term are all combined with an HMO product.

The *market diversification* dimension reflects the degree to which organizations are geographically concentrated or are spread across multiple markets (regional or national systems). Geographic proximity offers opportunities for coordination and consolidation that are, for the most part, unavailable in multimarket organizations. Many healthcare organizations are pursuing both single and multimarket strategies (viz., Columbia, Phycor, Aetna).

Implications for Information System Strategy

How do we apply the above framework to information system strategies? Table 3.2 provides examples of specific strategies that organizations can pursue, depending on the relative stability of their markets and their particular market and product strategies.

In stable market environments, most organizations tend to focus on the optimization of internal operations in order to maintain or increase market share by providing increased value to the customer (position strategy), or improve financial viability by improving internal operations (performance strategy). In such environments, information system strategies will tend to pursue purposes similar to overall organizational strategies. For example, hospitals may adopt order-entry result reporting technologies to improve internal operations.

In dynamic market environments, organizations tend to move more cautiously in building complex information systems, concentrating more on "essential" internal support and selectively on external support. With management much more engaged in assessing external markets and competitors, market intelligence systems can play a key role. Hospitals in dynamic markets, for example, will likely focus on developing physician linkages and referral technologies to shore up market share, but they may go slowly in building complex systems that integrate across physicians or tie them to their hospitals—at least until the market settles down and fluid physician/hospital partner relationships are clarified.

Internal systems may be used selectively to assist in developing external markets. For example, order-entry result reporting technologies could be adopted to assist physicians who wish to obtain patient diagnostic test results at their offices. Providing physician links not only improves internal operations, but also supports external market strategies. However, if the structure of relationships with physicians or the particular choices of partners are unsettled, such information system strategies would likely be pursued with caution.

The degree of service diversification influences the structure of information systems. Within horizontally expanded provider organizations, for example, information systems can be used to standardize production and delivery processes, production management systems, and managerial control systems. They also can integrate customer-oriented services through enterprise-wide referral, registration, and scheduling systems, thus enabling provider systems to act as single entities. In a more loosely structured alliance, however, investment in infrastructure support may be limited to only the highest priorities.

Because of diversity in service function and the need to integrate across businesses, vertically integrated systems require more complex clinical and financial information systems. For vertically integrated provider systems, greater challenges will come on the clinical side, given the diversity and planned interdependencies among clinical processes. Consolidated financial systems tend to be more standardized and therefore easier to develop. In general, the difficulties inherent in establishing and operating vertical strategies are duplicated in the im-

TABLE 3.2. Model for information system strategies

Business strategies		Stability of market structures	
Service diversification	Market diversification	Stable structure	Dynamic structure
Horizontally Integrated Systems (e.g., multiple acute care facilities)	Single Market	• Focus on optimization of operations • Integrated core clinical and financial transactional technologies • Standardization of technologies across facilities • Master patient index • Enterprise-wide scheduling and referral systems • Enterprise-wide financial control systems • Interfaced with physicians, insurance companies, and suppliers for optimizing internal operations • In-house systems vs. shared services	• Focus on flexibility and planning capabilities • Independent core clinical and financial transactional technologies • Do not invest in standardization across facilities • Master patient index • Flexible vs. proprietary technologies • Invest in turnkey operations when feasible • Enterprise-wide communication links • Enterprise-wide financial control systems • External communication linkages • External market and competitors' databases • Network competencies and interface engines • Shared services vs. in-house technologies
	Multiple Markets	Follow above strategies within each market with additional considerations: • Standardize technologies across services and facilities when economically feasible • Enterprise-wide financial control systems for the company • Centralize system selection processes • Decentralize system implementation processes • Centralize system evaluation processes	Follow above strategies within each market with additional considerations: • Do not invest in standardization of technologies unless economical feasible in the short term • Enterprise-wide financial control systems for the company • Decentralize system selection processes • Decentralize system implementation processes • Centralize system evaluation processes

TABLE 3.2. Model for information system strategies (*continued*)

Business strategies		Stability of market structures	
Service diversification	Market diversification	Stable structure	Dynamic structure
Vertically Integrated Systems (multiple facilities along continuum of care, e.g., diagnostic centers, clinics, acute care, home health care, nursing homes, etc.)	Single Market	Follow strategies for cell 1 above for acute care facilities. Additional considerations for vertically integrated services: • Standardize technologies across services and facilities when economically feasible and reduce costs of system maintenance and training • Enterprise-wide master patient index • Enterprise-wide communication links • Enterprise-wide financial control systems	Follow strategies for cell 2 above for acute care facilities. Additional considerations for vertically integrated services: • Do not invest in standardization of technologies unless economical feasible in the short term • Enterprise-wide master patient index • Enterprise-wide communication • Enterprise-wide financial control systems
	Multiple Markets	Follow strategies for cell 2 above for acute care facilities. Additional considerations for vertically integrated services: • Standardize technologies across services and facilities when economically feasible • Enterprise-wide master patient index within each market • Enterprise-wide communication links within each market • Enterprise-wide financial control systems for the company • Decentralize system selection processes • Decentralize system implementation processes • Centralize system evaluation processes	Follow strategies for cell 3 above for acute care facilities. Additional considerations for vertically integrated services: • Do not invest in standardization of technologies unless economical feasible in the short term • Enterprise-wide Master Patient Index within each market • Enterprise-wide communication links with each market • Enterprise-wide financial control systems for the company • Decentralize and standardize system selection processes • Decentralize system implementation processes • Centralize system evaluation processes with participation from affected facilities

plementation of supporting information systems. Such challenges are only exacerbated within dynamic market environments.

Differences in market diversification strategies have significant implications for the design of information systems. Local systems will be able to standardize clinical systems, for example, across geographically proximate facilities and providers. Regional and national systems may need to pursue local strategies for their local systems. Given the diversity of systems and environments at local market levels, however, such systems may need to move slowly in attempting to standardize information system strategies across markets.

In time, these regional and national systems may need to invest in interface engines and technologies for standardization. Technologies like Health Level 7 (HL7) can greatly assist in developing standard data across markets, thus facilitating the development of decision support and comparative financial reporting systems within a multimarket structure. Multimarket systems may also need to invest in data warehousing capabilities to develop clinical databases from clinical transactional technologies. This would facilitate the development of clinical performance assessments, including national and regional benchmarking of clinical outcomes, which could help improve quality and reduce the cost of care.

One of the needs of multimarket healthcare organizations is to develop communication links among facilities for administrative, clinical, and educational purposes. This may be easier to accomplish for local than for regional or national systems—and the rationale for such linkages would, of course, be far stronger. Local systems can install their own networks to transfer financial as well as confidential clinical data from one facility to another through secured communication lines, a strategy that is less feasible for regional and national systems. The World Wide Web and the Internet make it possible to link facilities beyond local environments, but these linkages are on public lines and thus lack adequate security. This is why many regional systems are now looking to alternatives like banking and other proprietary networks for solutions to system networking.

Strategy Markers for Information Systems

By way of summary, we conclude with four strategy markers that organizations might wish to consider when assessing their information system strategies in the context of market and strategic realities.

- **Incrementalism.** With respect to information systems, this safe strategy means that organizations break their decisions into parts, prioritize them, and then make decisions over time, gradually and successively. Information systems may be seen as providing much-needed integration across multiproduct and multimarket companies. But the problems in building integrated systems are many and complex, and information systems simply do not address many of the critical structural and leadership problems inherent in building complicated delivery systems. Therefore, given the costs of building information systems and the ever-changing technologies, it is important that executives time their investments in information systems, allowing for critical organizational and strategic decisions and arrangements to be made first. It is too easy for organizations to be persuaded by flimsy arguments that "two or three birds can be killed with one stone." There is a strong need for organizations to conduct careful assessments of their market environments, establish clear priorities in information system design, and implement their decisions incrementally and at a pace that is consistent with their market conditions and particular strategies.
- **Standardization.** Acquisition of highly unique, untested, and proprietary information systems may introduce levels of risk that outweigh the promised ben-

efits. Thus, in periods of change, there is a great need for standards to evolve in system design and performance. Until they do, healthcare organizations will need to be cautious when investing in information systems. This could lead, for example, to outsourcing strategies where feasible, holding off on internal acquisitions until such standards are established in the field.

- **Interfaces and internal controls.** Often the demand for systems that link and facilitate interorganizational coordination and control are driven by overestimates of market change and premature projections of consolidation and system integration. In today's environment, healthcare executives must make careful and realistic assessments of integration strategies, giving priority to those areas where the returns to integration can be documented. Again, this points up the need for caution when investing in information system infrastructure within complex multiorganizational structures, especially under conditions of environmental uncertainty and change.
- **Institutionalization and rigidities.** Limitations in information system strategies can often produce critical bottlenecks that forestall the implementation of an organization's strategies. On the other hand, early investments in information systems can themselves become "institutionalized," thereby introducing rigidities in organizations that slow the adoption of important market strategies arising out of changing market conditions. Therefore, it is essential that information system strategy be carefully aligned with an organization's overall strategic framework.

Clearly, there needs to be close coordination between information and organizational strategies. This is as true in health care as it is in any other industry. It should be remembered, however, that *the strategic agendas of most organizations are necessarily idealistic.* They are conceptual. They are based in the assumptions held by leaders of organizations and the field in general. As such, they are often in error and intermittently modified, even more so in uncertain and turbulent times.

Clearly, there should be no single strategy guiding information system investments in this industry. Each organization is unique. The many strategic and operational issues should be weighed in the context of individual organizational capabilities, structures, and strategies. Organizations vary importantly by how stable their environments are, their degree and form of product/service diversification, and whether they are in single or multiple markets. Therefore, like all other major investments, information system strategies should be measured ultimately by the costs and benefits they are estimated to generate, given the particulars of individual organizations and their markets.

Finally, we emphasize once again that information system investments should be carefully timed and sequenced. If well-timed, they can provide significant, often unmatched (in the short term, at least) competitive advantages. Mistimed, they can easily reverse hard-earned gains in market position, even interfere with an organization's ability to maneuver strategically. In the end, it all comes back to the vision *and* the analytic capabilities of an organization's leadership. If they get it right, they win. If not, they learn valuable lessons about both market competition and the vagaries of information system strategy.

References

Amburgey, T.L. and A.S. Miner. 1989. "Strategic Momentum: The Effects of Repetitive, Positional, and Contextual Momentum on Merger Activity." *Strategic Management Journal* 10(5): 413–430.

Collis, D.J. and C.A. Montgomery. 1995. "Competing on Resources: Strategy in the 1990s." *Harvard Business Review,* July–August: 118–128.

Cringely, R.X. 1996. *Accidental Empires: How the Boys of Silicon Valley Make Their Millions, Battle Foreign Competition, and Still Can't Get a Date.* New York: Harper Business.

D'Aveni, R.A. 1994. *Hypercompetition: Managing the Dynamics of Strategic Maneuvering.* New York: The Free Press.

Gates, B. 1995. *The Road Ahead.* New York: Viking Penguin.

Harrigan, K. 1985. *Strategic Flexibility: A Management Guide for Changing Times.* Lexington, Mass.: Lexington Books.

InterStudy. 1994. *InterStudy's Competitive Edge.* Minneapolis, Minn.: InterStudy.

Jager, R.D. and R. Ortiz. 1997. *In the Company of Giants: Candid Conversations with the Visionaries of the Digital World.* New York: McGraw-Hill.

Miles, R.E. and C.C. Snow. 1978. *Organizational Strategy, Structure, and Process.* New York: McGraw-Hill.

Mintzberg, H. 1990. "Strategy Formulation: Schools of Thought," in *Perspectives on Strategic Management,* ed J. Frederickson. Boston: Ballinger.

Mintzberg, H. 1994. *The Rise and Fall of Strategic Planning: Reconceiving Roles for Planning, Plans, Planners.* New York: Free Press.

Porter, M.E. 1996. "What Is Strategy?" *Harvard Business Review,* November/December: 61–78.

Quigley, J.V. 1993. *Vision: How Leaders Can Develop It, Share It, and Sustain It.* New York: McGraw-Hill.

Wallace, J. 1997. *Overdrive: Bill Gates and the Race to Control Cyberspace.* New York: John Wiley & Sons.

Part 2

Transformational Processes

4

Planning for Performance

RICHARD N. KRAMER AND JUDITH V. DOUGLAS

The rate of change in health care is not abating. Integrated delivery networks are addressing issues of access and cross-continuum care management, and identifying emerging technologies that will support best practices. Competition continues to be fierce, demanding top-level performance and operational effectiveness.

As we enter a period of increased spending on information technology (IT), strategic planning is assuming renewed significance, following the pattern of the early 1980s, when IT spending was peaking. Today the pace is faster and the competition fiercer—old models don't work.

The Model

To respond to the pressing needs of healthcare organizations, First Consulting Group has developed a new approach to strategic information management planning. Known as SIMP, it differs markedly from traditional planning models in philosophy, approach, and, most importantly, in results. To date, SIMP has been used in a variety of settings; for each engagement, the approach was tailored to address specific needs. The results? Tighter alignment between business strategy and IT strategy, a better understanding of risk and return on investment, tools that reflect best practices and increase operational effectiveness, and ultimately a pragmatic, implementable plan.

Business-Driven

The overriding difference between SIMP and earlier approaches is this: SIMP focuses on improving *operational* performance. When organizations select customer intimacy as their key differentiator, the first task is to identify and differentiate those process that are considered to be strategic and seek to focus investment in those processes, not simply in information technology. SIMP begins by identifying and aligning the business goals with supporting processes to drive information management needs. The intent is to build the essential infrastructure and acquire support for high-priority enterprise business strategies. Investments in information systems are based on enterprise-level business decisions, not aggregated technology "wish lists."

This focus on the business of health care transforms the planning process. With SIMP, information technology—along with changes in processes and organization—is implemented as an information management initiative. From the outset, the planning process is structured to accommodate uncertainty about future payer demands, competition, and organizational strategies. Above all, the SIMP model requires the willing and active participation of key executives and clinical leaders who understand the importance of information management in the planning process. Developed and continuously updated to address today's competitive marketplace, SIMP appeals to these executives and the organizations they serve. *Acknowledging rapid change, SIMP compresses planning time frames and targets the development of concise action plans, not massive planning reports.*

Knowledge-Based

Driven by the business strategy and stated in business terms, the SIMP process brings new insights provided by applied research in healthcare organizations and by targeted studies of ambulatory systems, clinical data repositories, and Internet applications. Comparative data on best practices, such as that developed by First Consulting Group in its study of 10 organizations (see Table 4.1), can help integrated delivery networks move "beyond the bottom line" and focus on what information management can contribute to the continuum of care (*Modern Healthcare* 1997). The SIMP model draws on and adds to these knowledge bases.

Knowledge transfer is critical to the analysis of alternative business and environmental scenarios. *To succeed in a rapidly changing industry, healthcare organizations must draw upon new knowledge while simultaneously leveraging their staff's knowledge of the installed base and current performance.* This requires repeated and rigorous challenges to the thinking involved in the planning process. To ensure that these do occur, SIMP includes a series of formal work-

TABLE 4.1. Integrated delivery networks in FCG study of best practices.

Organizations studied
HealthSystem Minnesota, Minneapolis
Henry Ford Health System, Detroit
Integris Health, Oklahoma City
Intermountain Health Care, Salt Lake City
North Mississippi Health Services, Tupelo
Partners HealthCare System, Boston
ProMedica Health Systems, Toledo
Providence Health System, Portland
Sentara Health System, Norfolk
University Medical Center, Tucson

shops in which meaningful dialogue among leadership is facilitated and the thought process is continually challenged. These workshops help promote understanding at all levels of the organization—and obtain buy-in from key stakeholders.

Fast-Tracked

The SIMP model is designed to support a fast-tracked process. The core planning team is deliberately kept small, and its members include senior-level leaders and physicians. Rather than beginning with a time-consuming survey of multiple constituencies and users, the team starts with the organization's strategic direction. The project team is composed to leverage existing teams within the organization, and the project leader is a "business unit neutral" person. A comprehensive communications plan offsets the lack of broad input.

The consultants draw upon their prior work and industry knowledge to provide a starter set of models. These are reviewed and adapted, and the organization's vision is documented in a series of future information models. To keep the process on the fast track, strategy development and tactical rollout overlap. Migration plans are identified to redesign process, align the organization, and implement IT infrastructure and applications over a two- to three-year horizon. As consensus needs are identified, the team targets "quick hits" and launches strategic infrastructure "now" projects. The time frame for action is compressed, and detailed planning is deferred until funding is determined.

Throughout, the core team targets initiatives that are practical, affordable, focused on key issues, and understandable—in a word, implementable.

The Methodology

The word "implementable" is key. In a competitive environment, performance counts; healthcare institutions cannot afford to plan without achieving timely results and reaching measurable goals. Given the impossibility of doing everything everywhere, the question is where to focus on the "big win" and where to make incremental improvements to stay in the game. The SIMP model focuses on both and offers clear guides to decision making. SIMPS's distinctive fast tracking—including quick hits and "now" projects—targets incremental gains. The bottom line: *If planning doesn't improve performance, it has failed.*

Understand Tools and Templates

SIMP offers a proven methodology, complete with specially designed templates and tools, that makes fast tracking close to risk-free and validates decisions through a rigorous "challenge" process. The templates provide valuable comparisons to relevant industry standards and best practices, while the tools help delineate, focus, and monitor projects, as well as measure progress. Both serve to advance the planning model and keep it understandable at all levels of the organization by making it and its component activities explicit and identifiable to the participants. Both are continually refined and recalibrated for optimal functionality in a fast-changing environment.

Under the SIMP approach, the core planning team has the option to adopt these tool sets "as is" or to modify them. Like the knowledge base, the tool set stands assembled, updated, validated, and ready for use. State-of-the-art templates and tools make it possible to focus on business issues, not seek out or create planning methodologies. In many ways, SIMP is like the state-of-the-art, off-the-shelf software that has replaced in-house custom-built solutions: it offers optimal functionality in the shortest time and at the lowest cost.

Plan Phases

As shown in Figure 4.1, the model includes seven phases that proceed in a stream of activities, some of which overlap. This overlapping is critical to fast tracking while redesigning key business processes. SIMP delineates each phase in detail, guiding the core planning group and other participants through the process and ensuring that key elements and activities are not overlooked. These phases can be grouped in three clusters—launch effort, develop models, and deliver strategy. Major milestones are reached along the way, and participants address key components in structured workshops, using materials and methodologies provided by SIMP.

Launch Effort

- **Initiate project.** The first phase differs from traditional planning kickoffs in its emphasis on tailoring the planning process to ensure that the model is adjusted to meet the needs of the enterprise. Equal weight is placed on establishing expectations and confirming them with key executives. To fast-track the project launch, SIMP provides templates to help in key areas—for example, putting together the core project team, developing communications plans and charter statements, and completing a project work plan with milestones and measurable outputs.

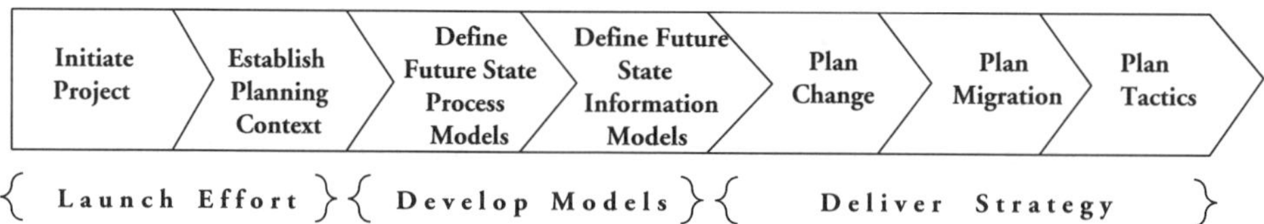

FIGURE 4.1. The Seven Phases of Strategic Information Management Planning
© FCG 1998

- **Establish planning context.** This second phase seeks agreement on issues defining the context in which planning will occur. These include environmental assumptions, business strategies (both baseline and alternative), current situation, and magnitude of change. Focused on performance improvement, this phase elicits executive team input to help target business processes, success measures, and likely changes. The projected results include alignment of business strategy with major processes, along with fact-based understanding of the challenges ahead and the level of change required. Here, knowledge of best practices across the industry adds value.

Develop Models

- **Define future state business process model.** This phase targets tailoring business process models to develop a "future map" and document current and desired future states. Working with the process design team, the core planning group confirms business processes for key strategic initiatives, down to the subprocess level. To ensure that the plan is business-driven and implementable, the teams define metrics, classify current performance, and identify gaps. The results? A model that depicts future state business processes, implications for change, and "now" projects related to key processes.
- **Define future state information management model.** This phase involves creating a concrete representation of the future information management direction. In addition to confirming the current status of information management (including gaps) and reviewing future models, the core planning and process design teams identify core infrastructure needs and develop infrastructure, organizational, and applications models. Then, identifying key information management issues, they test models against scenarios. The rigor of these efforts extends to a formal challenge process, validating the models developed and reaffirming consensus on priority issues and projects.

Deliver Strategy

- **Plan change.** The first of the last three phases in planning for strategy rollout, this phase targets agreement on high-value, high-priority change initiatives and an assessment of risks and alternative scenarios. Participants define initiatives that deliver baseline infrastructure, achieve business performance objectives, and confirm current workload and capital demand. Change projects are prioritized, and existing projects are evaluated for modification, deferral, or shutdown. To prepare to manage risks, this phase brings in the executive team and external challengers, continuing and concluding the rigor of the formal challenge process. Results are the prioritized change projects, including the identification and initiation of quick hits and "now" projects related to the change agenda.
- **Plan migration.** This phase defines major activities, schedules, the order of magnitude of resource requirements, and the expected value of planned projects. Activities include sequencing projects and their prerequisites, summariz-

ing results, and developing educational and marketing materials. The resulting migration plan states macrolevel costs and schedule estimates—both are key in monitoring implementation and measuring progress. To help avert risk, a watch list itemizes events that trigger alternative scenarios.

- **Plan tactics.** Under SIMP's fast tracking, this final phase includes tactical planning for "now" projects and occurs concurrent with strategy. It allows the planning organization to initiate high-value, high-priority projects as soon as possible, rolling out "quick hits" and gaining immediate benefits. At the same time, the plan is in the approval process. This approach differentiates SIMP from earlier planning models and provides the opportunity to aggressively educate stakeholders and gain buy-in. Comprehensive tactical planning remains a follow-up activity, after the plan is approved and funding identified.

SIMP at Work in an Integrated Delivery Network

Consider the use of the SIMP model in an integrated delivery network (IDN). This IDN (let's call it AllCare) is rapidly moving toward a market that Shortell identifies as Stage 4, or a Strict Managed Care "Value" Market, with a high level of integration (Shortell et al. 1996, pp. 32–33). AllCare has strong relationships with insurers and community-based services and holds a majority share in the regional market, but it has work to do in the areas of wellness, clinical integration, outcomes, and population-based and community health. These have clear implications for its information management plan components and timing for implementation.

In establishing the planning context, AllCare identifies environmental drivers. With a population that is 65 percent Medicare, AllCare has a vested interest in maintaining the community health status. Demands are increasing for alternative delivery models with lower-cost ambulatory care that offers improved clinical effectiveness. Resentful independent specialists constitute a challenge in the areas of physician integration and incentive alignment. For-profit practice management entities and urban megasystems pose competitive threats. A new Medicare product promises a spike in enrollment that will have to be managed, and AllCare is hoping to achieve a critical mass of membership.

Where does AllCare stand compared to other IDNs? As Figure 4.2 illustrates, a look at the 21st century integration survey of over 40 established IDNs indicates their level of integration in four key areas. Integration in the information and clinical areas lags behind structural and operational integration. As a mid-later stage IDN, AllCare is broadening its focus from patients to members and on to populations. This incurs new risks and has implications for information management.

How should AllCare move forward? Their purpose is to develop a business-process based plan that will enable them to do so, through a blend of organization, process improvement, and information management. They target aggressive

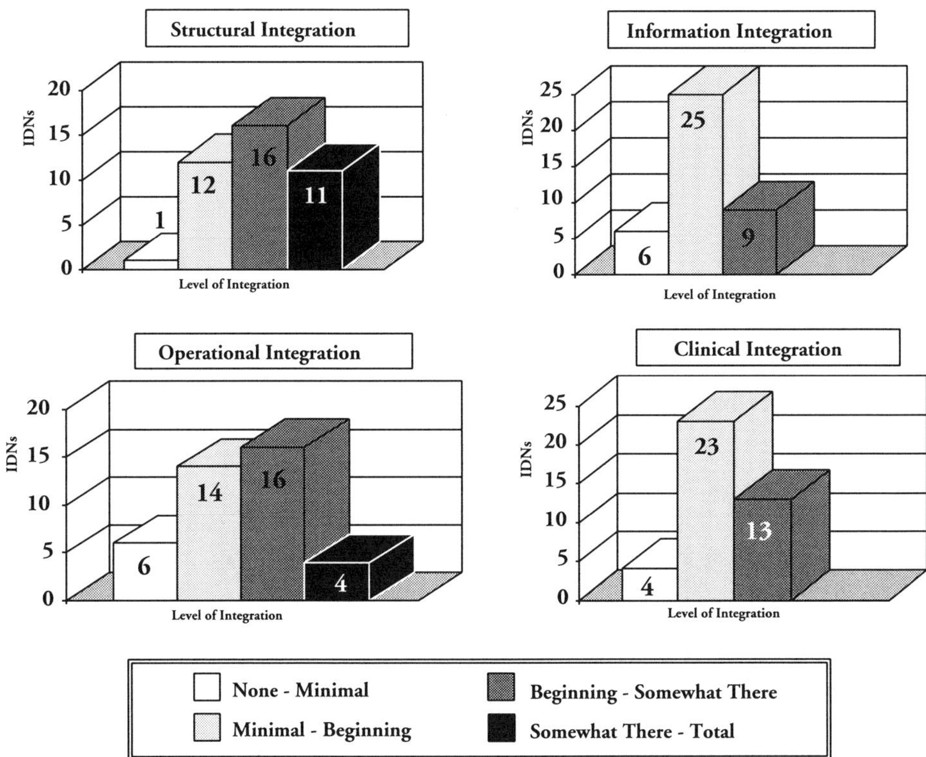

FIGURE 4.2. IDN Integration in Four Key Areas
© Copyright FCG 1997

growth in managed care and intend to leverage data as a strategic asset, relying on common systems and existing investments where possible.

The immediate challenge is to define the future state business model and the future state information model—the two middle phases under SIMP. Because they, like many other healthcare institutions, do not have a framework for process definitions in place, AllCare's subject matter experts work with the process model provided as a template, tailoring it to their own special circumstances and corporate culture. To extend AllCare's knowledge base, external subject matter experts are brought in to share emerging models.

Both phases are rigorous, requiring that the core planning and process design teams develop a "future map" and create a concrete representation of the future information management direction for their institution. Here, AllCare conducts a gap analysis, identifying the implications of the business processes on their network architecture and pinpointing any potential gaps in the ability of the current network to enable the business processes.

These phases include a formal challenge process involving some forthright and hard-hitting discussions. Though the experience is intense at times, it results in true consensus. AllCare develops a new process model, aligning strategies and requirements to the core processes they identify.

As the AllCare team members work, they "map" core processes to subprocesses, applications, information/integration tools, and infrastructure. For example, the team maps access to care to wellness/disease management protocols, rules-based clinical protocols, administrative and clinical warehouses, and enterprise messaging. They assess current status, suggest incremental improvements, and identify advanced models. For example, they suggest leveraging existing databases in support of managed care contracting, now largely manual for physicians, as an interim solution while working toward full integration of contract management with other systems.

To plan for strategy rollout, AllCare brings the executive team back into the planning meetings and calls in external challengers to keep the process rigorous. At decision-making time, the team must ask several crucial questions. What offers high value? What level of support does the initiative in question have? Is it doable, affordable, durable, urgent? What priority does it merit? What are the risks associated with doing it right now, doing it later, or not doing it at all? Ultimately, the AllCare strategy adopts each of these three options.

For the short term, the team decides to phase out the legacy system, while completing the network infrastructure and desktop migration already budgeted. Over the next three years, they will improve their three core processes—access to care, provision of care, and population health management. These processes are where they, as members of a maturing IDN, can make the "big win." Their focus on access to care ranges from enrollment and eligibility to member financial management. Information management initiatives—for example, a new health plan system and a new physician and ambulatory system—will support not only access but also the other core processes.

The AllCare team's migration strategy for access to care involves such activities as defining and rolling out enterprise registration and scheduling standards. The team also plans to leverage and integrate these with the call center's enterprise scheduling capabilities. To keep on the fast track, AllCare team members make a first cut at estimating costs as they sequence projects, and they initiate quick hits and immediate priority strategic projects as the strategic plan moves through the approval process. They decide to tackle comprehensive tactical planning on their own, following the SIMP model of tying their spreadsheets to their strategic plan by attaching yearly and total costs to each process.

Successful Planning

For AllCare, says one of its top executives, the SIMP process helped uncover common ground and improve understanding of enterprise issues—an understanding critical to any maturing IDN. *We believe the success of the process resulted in part from its pragmatic, business-oriented approach.* Rapidly distinguishing strategic processes and aggressively pursued "now" projects gave the planning credibility. Following a formal model ensured that assumptions and implications were made explicit, challenged, validated, and always linked to key business initiatives.

Other Settings, Other Challenges

First Consulting Group has used the SIMP approach successfully with other organizations. In New England, for example, we worked with an IDN to develop an information plan that would allow them to respond to managed care and build differentiated services. At the same time, the IDN was merging two hospitals—and integrating multiple physician practices and hospital systems. The outcomes were favorable. Their executive team set priorities based on business needs and sold the plan to key constituencies. Before the planning process was through, they had launched projects to strengthen their network architecture, build an application infrastructure, and respond to urgent priorities.

Because the SIMP approach can be tailored to the specifics of each organization, it can address a variety of circumstances. For one healthcare organization that had developed a list of information management projects exceeding their available resources, the process allowed them to backpedal, linking information projects to key business initiatives and developing prioritization criteria. The result was a migration plan for implementing priority information investments within the organization's budgetary constraints—evidence of the flexibility that SIMP provides.

This flexibility supports the development of plans of varying scopes, including truly massive efforts. Intent on linking their information plan to their business, a multistate Blue Cross/Blue Shield organization developed a migration plan incorporating 14 strategic projects and identifying 8 to 10 more for future consideration.

Finally, the SIMP approach improves the odds with highly demanding constituencies. Consider engagements involving physicians in ambulatory care settings, where communication is difficult from the start. Here, the model has succeeded in eliminating barriers to progress by building communication to all constituencies into the process.

The Value Proposition

Our experiences to date confirm the value of the SIMP approach. Business-driven, knowledge-based, and fast-tracked, it does what traditional planning models failed to do. Tied to results, it sets forth measurable goals. Pragmatic, it considers immediate needs and requirements for durability and flexibility in changing markets, including issues of affordability and "do-ability." In a move that wins over constituent groups and rewards executive commitment, *it acts to meet immediate needs immediately, within the context of ongoing planning.* At a time when organizational and technical networking both support and demand collaboration, it is collaborative, actively recruiting new insights and outside knowledge bases.

With SIMP, planning is a rigorous process, one that considers alternative scenarios and is formally challenged before adoption. It is not a leisurely exercise that produces fat reports. It is a tightly focused process that results in a pragmatic, implementable plan that aligns IT with an enterprise's goals and direction.

References

Morrissey, J. 1997. "Getting Beyond the Bottom Line." *Modern Healthcare* 127(26): 112–118.

Shortell, S.M., R.R. Gillies, D.A. Anderson, K.M. Erickson, and J.B. Mitchell. 1996. *Remaking Health Care in America: Building Organized Delivery Systems*. San Francisco: Jossey-Bass.

5

Enterprise Information Architecture

Tom Hurley and Donald Tompkins

For the past decade, organizations have been obsessed with the notion of aligning information technology (IT) with their business processes. Although this seems like an intrinsic good in theory, evidence suggests that such investments rarely fulfilled expectations. Organizations spent billions of dollars on IT in the 1980s and 1990s; few of them, however, have realized significant benefit from their investment.

The problem with alignment seems to stem from organizations' failure to keep up with changes in the business drivers. As Peter Keen (1991, p. 211) said: "[Aligning business and technology] is not about managing change, it is about taking charge of change. . . . The key to alignment is *relationships*, not strategy." In health care, the investment in IT as a percent of the operating budget has been significantly less than in industry in general—typically on the order of 2 percent or less (HPHIMSS Survey 1997). Still, the challenge in health care to leverage the huge volumes of data into useful information—and more importantly, into knowledge—is greater than in any other industry. William Inmon observed:

> Knowledge will become one of the distinguishing assets of successful companies. . . . Knowledge entails the synthesis of information to provide a corporate entity with an improved awareness and understanding of itself, its human and other resources, and its business environment. (1997, p. xv)

The process of turning data into information and information into knowledge requires *aligning* and *linking* information systems to the business processes. Aligning information systems to the business processes of health care (e.g., delivering care, managing care) requires an in-depth understanding of the linkage between business process and information to support those processes. Just as important—and just as difficult to quantify—is the way in which those business processes relate to the other business processes within the enterprise.

The recent trends in interface engines and data warehouses are an attempt to address this problem without requiring massive changes in the legacy information systems. Most of these data warehouse efforts, however, are designed for a limited information need (e.g., retrospective analysis of a few high-expense care protocols). These approaches do not address the change required to improve operational processes, which is where the real benefit of information systems can be realized.

As healthcare organizations try to tackle more complex problems like those surrounding the access to care process, data warehouses and interface engines will not be enough. Healthcare organizations will need to take a more holistic and integrated view of their business processes and their information requirements. Enterprise information architecture (EIA) is one methodology for linking information systems to business process.

Historical Perspective: The Zachman Framework

In the late 1980s, John Zachman, who was then a member of IBM's Business Strategy Group, published a landmark paper on information systems architecture in the *IBM Systems Journal* (Zachman 1987). "A Framework for Information Systems Architecture" outlined a methodology for defining the interdependencies between business strategy and information strategy using an architecture analogy. His methodology was easy to use—and, more importantly, easy to understand. Now known as the "Zachman framework" (Zachman Institute for Framework Advancement), his principles have become the foundation for many new enterprise-wide IT planning methodologies, including EIA.

Zachman believed that in order to move from "chaos to order and structure" in information systems, an architectural approach to information systems planning is necessary. Each stage in the building of a house requires different levels of detail. At each stage, decisions need to be made about what materials comprise the product, how it will work, where the components are located, who is involved, when tasks needed to be completed, and why they are important. In the Zachman framework, the who, what, when, where, and why translate into equivalent information abstractions: data, function, network, people, time, and motivation.

Zachman subdivided the building process into five stages or perspectives, each adding clarification and detail to its predecessor. These five perspectives—planner, owner, designer, builder, and subcontractor—closely interacted with his information abstractions. By creating a matrix where the perspectives were the rows and the abstractions were the columns, he was able to create a simple graphical representation of the key artifacts and relationships that make up an enterprise's information needs and solutions. The representation is easily understood by both the technical and business communities, and it clearly shows that information systems map to business processes, not to technology.

The Zachman framework itself is simply that, a framework. It provides an overview of the process that an enterprise should go through in order to maximize IT capabilities. As Figure 5.1 illustrates, the total framework itself fits on a single page, and each "cell" in the framework represents its own architecture.

Since the inception of the Zachman framework, a number of highly detailed methodologies, or architectures, have been developed around a single perspective or abstraction (the intersection of a perspective and abstraction is usually defined as an architecture). Enterprise information architecture, which will soon be

A FRAMEWORK FOR ENTERPRISE ARCHITECTURE™

	DATA *What*	FUNCTION *How*	NETWORK *Where*	PEOPLE *Who*	TIME *When*	MOTIVATION *Why*	
SCOPE (CONTEXTUAL) *Planner*	List of Things Important to the Business ENTITY = Class of Business Thing	List of Processes the Business Performs Function = Class of Business Process	List of Locations in which the Business Operates Node = Major Business Location	List of Organizations Important to the Business People = Major Organizations	List of Events Significant to the Business Time = Major Business Event	List of Business Goals/Strat Ends/Means=Major Bus. Goal/ Critical Success Factor	SCOPE (CONTEXTUAL) *Planner*
ENTERPRISE MODEL (CONCEPTUAL) *Owner*	e.g. Semantic Model Ent = Business Entity Reln = Business Relationship	e.g. Business Process Model Proc. = Business Process I/O = Business Resources	e.g. Logistics Network Node = Business Location Link = Business Linkage	e.g. Work Flow Model People = Organization Unit Work = Work Product	e.g. Master Schedule Time = Business Event Cycle = Business Cycle	e.g. Business Plan End = Business Objective Means = Business Strategy	ENTERPRISE MODEL (CONCEPTUAL) *Owner*
SYSTEM MODEL (LOGICAL) *Designer*	e.g. Logical Data Model Ent = Data Entity Reln = Data Relationship	e.g. "Application Architecture" Proc .= Application Function I/O = User Views	e.g. "Distributed System Architecture" Node = I/S Function (Processor, Storage, etc) Link = Line Characteristics	e.g. Human Interface Architecture People = Role Work = Deliverable	e.g. Processing Structure Time = System Event	e.g., Business Rule Model End = Structural Assertion Means =Action Assertion	SYSTEM MODEL (LOGICAL) *Designer*
TECHNOLOGY MODEL (PHYSICAL) *Builder*	e.g. Physical Data Model Ent = Segment/Table/etc. Reln = Pointer/Key/etc.	e.g. "System Design" Proc.= Computer Function I/O = Screen/Device Formats	e.g. "System Architecture" Node = Hardware/System Software Link = Line Specifications	e.g. Presentation Architecture People = User Work = Screen Format	e.g. Control Structure Cycle = Component Cycle	e.g. Rule Design Means = Action	TECHNOLOGY CONSTRAINED MODEL (PHYSICAL) *Builder*
DETAILED REPRESEN-TATIONS (OUT-OF-CONTEXT) *Sub-Contractor*	e.g. Data Definition Ent = Field Reln = Address	e.g. "Program" Proc.= Language Stmt I/O = Control Block	e.g. "Network Architecture" Node = Addresses Link = Protocols	People=Identity Work=Job	e.g. Timing Definition Time=Interrupt Cycle=Machine Cycle	e.g. Rule Specification End=Sub-Condition Means=Step	DETAILED REPRESEN-TATIONS (OUT-OF CONTEXT) *Sub-Contractor*
FUNCTIONING ENTERPRISE	e.g. DATA	e.g. FUNCTION	e.g. NETWORK	e.g. ORGANIZATION	e.g. SCHEDULE	e.g. STRATEGY	FUNCTIONING ENTERPRISE

FIGURE 5.1. The Zachman framework. Data reprinted with permission from John A. Zachman, Zachman International.

discussed in detail, is a methodology focusing on Zachman's top two perspectives, planner and owner.

Architecture: Concept and Characteristics

Architecture is not a new concept in software engineering. In the 1950s and 1960s, COBOL (COmmon Business Oriented Language) was developed as a standard so it would run on different types of computers. System architects, the original practitioners of software architecture, focused their engineering talents on the infrastructure of the system to ensure that all its pieces worked together efficiently. In the beginning, system architects focused exclusively on three types of architectures: system, application, and network. The system architecture defined how major components of the system (like hardware and operating systems) worked together, the application architecture defined how applications would be developed to use the system architecture, and the network architecture defined how physically separated hardware components would communicate with each other.

Although data architecture was not originally a separate architecture (it was usually a part of the system and application architectures), its importance in today's system designs has created a whole new field of data architecture. In the past ten years, largely because of the Zachman framework, the term "architecture" has taken on a much broader meaning. Today, a legitimate architecture should have most, if not all, of the following characteristics:

- Information systems implementations should reflect the characteristics of the business.
- Data should be consistent from application to application.
- Hardware/systems software should be compatible from end-to-end.
- Business rules should be enforced consistently across implementations.
- Systems should be defined logically, independent of technology constraints.
- Change should be incorporated as a design criterion.

In addition, a usable architecture should contain two levels of abstraction: the blueprint and the specification. The blueprint should be a high-level overview of the architecture that is easy to read, identifies at a high level the key elements and relationships, and helps the reader locate components in the detailed specification. This specification must contain enough detail to meet the six requirements identified in the above list.

Components of Enterprise Information Architecture

The EIA model is actually a collection of six architectures that integrate the enterprise's key processes with the information requirements needed to support them. Four of these architectures—data, process, application, and technology—

have been established as part of the EIA model. The two other architectures discussed in this section, knowledge and integration, identify critical components of an enterprise's information systems that are in addition to the classical model.

Data Architecture

One of the many ironies of the information age is that most of today's information systems produce very little information. They do, however, produce staggering amounts of data. Data is one of the most concrete components of information systems; it is easy to see, manipulate, and package. As stated before, though, data is not information. Information is the product of knowledge, and knowledge is poorly represented in today's information systems.

Still, even if data is not information, it remains a critical component of an enterprise's information system. Ever since the creation of graphic methodologies to represent units of data and their relationships to each other, data architecture has been a popular way to represent systems. Unlike the classical data model, defined as part of the information engineering process, a data architecture that is part of an EIA is clearly defined in the context of the business processes that use it.

Though the data architecture is important to the EIA, an enterprise must not allow it to overshadow the other architectures simply because it is the easiest to understand and represent. After all, the current data architectures eventually will be replaced with object architecture. Although the promise of objects has been long in coming, the basic premise—that an object is both the data and the actions one can perform on the data—is the natural outcome of today's evolving information engineering.

Process Architecture

The process architecture identifies the enterprise's key business activities. Most of the information required to develop this application should already exist in the enterprise's strategic business plan; if a strategic plan does not exist, then there is little reason to continue developing the EIA. Assuming the strategic plan is written and does have a definition of key business activities, the next step is to dissect these activities and define their functional components. This process should continue until all the key processes are defined.

The level of dissection should be decided at the onset of EIA implementation—if required, it can iterate down to a set of very specific tasks. Once the dissection has reached the agreed-upon level, each subprocess needs to be mapped to the functional area of the organization that performs the process. At this point in the EIA process, it is not practical to correct any overlaps or gaps in the processes, since this would have a significant impact on the organization and is not part of the EIA's scope. It is, however, important to highlight the overlaps and gaps for future planning.

Application Architecture

The application architecture defines the applications that support key business activities defined in the process architecture. The term "application" suggests a logical grouping of functions that support specific business needs like patient accounting, pharmacy, radiology, and managed care. Until recently, applications were designed exclusively to support the specific needs of a single department. Of course, the problem with these departmental systems is that a department is not an enterprise; an enterprise is a seamless integration of departments. This leads to the logical conclusion that departmental systems must be integrated to better support the enterprise.

In health care today, the integration of departmental systems usually has meant developing interfaces between systems. For example, most departmental systems require admission/discharge/transfer (ADT) system information in order to verify orders that are being placed on their system. Without an ADT interface to the other departments, the patient must be continually readmitted, thereby creating a collection of unique patient identifiers throughout the enterprise. Even though many individual organizations have solved this multiple patient ID, the new reality of healthcare consolidation is creating problems for the patient index. Even though healthcare organizations have been trying to integrate applications with interfaces, the need to look at application functionality across the enterprise is still a critical part of the EIA.

Technology Architecture

Even though the primary focus of the enterprise information architecture is on the enterprise's business needs, technology still has a major impact on how those needs will be accomplished and how much it will cost. The technology architecture documents the enterprise's current use of information technologies, as well as the new technologies that will be required to meet the future needs of the business. Technology here includes such infrastructure components as mainframes, midrange, client server, end-user devices, networks (local and wide area), network operating systems, and development tools. (For a more complete discussion of technological possibilities, see Chapter 13.)

Integration Architecture

Systems integration has become a popular IT strategy in the '90s. Its popularity, along with the complexity and necessity of integrating systems, is why the integration architecture is a necessary part of the enterprise information architecture. Before describing the specific format of the integration architecture, it will be helpful to define the seven levels of integration.

- **Level 1—interfaces.** These involve the transportation of data between multiple systems. Most major healthcare systems are interfaced today; however, many are still point-to-point with very little integrity. In the past five years, most large enterprises have moved to interface engines in order to reduce the permutations of point-to-point interfaces they had to maintain.

- **Level 2—network integration.** This type of integration connects many systems and users electronically. The most popular form of network integration is local area networks. Internets and Intranets are also becoming very popular for employees and customers who cannot connect locally.
- **Level 3—workgroup integration.** This is a way to connect groups of users to facilitate group communication. The most common form of workgroup integration is e-mail, though the World Wide Web is also becoming a popular way for corporations to disseminate information to employees and customers.
- **Level 4—data integration.** This allows an enterprise to move data from multiple systems into a common data view or model. This type of integration has become very popular recently due to concepts like data warehousing, data marts, data mining, and decision support. The biggest problem with data integration is keeping both the data content and context current, a task that can require tremendous effort.
- **Level 5—application integration.** This connects multiple applications so they can share each other's data, processing, connections, and resources. The popularity and growth of the middleware industry, responsible for such products as remote procedure calls, e-mail, object request broker, stored procedures, and queuing, testify to how important this form of integration is to the enterprise. It is also a testament to the aphorism, "the cure is worse than the disease." Today, the middleware market is still highly fragmented, proprietary, and specialized, and no single solution works in all cases.
- **Level 6—object integration.** This allows multiple applications to reuse common object components. In the past five years, however, companies that have built new systems or replaced old systems have been using object technology. Though the first round of object projects did not leverage the advantages of reusability, encapsulation, and polymorphism, many lessons have been learned. The time is right to create true modular software that can be used in hundreds of applications across the enterprise.
- **Level 7—plenary integration.** As the term implies, this is integration that is complete in every way. A good example of plenary integration is the human body. Not only is each major system fully integrated (e.g., heart, veins, blood cells), each system also is fully integrated with every other system. Developing an EIA is the first step in achieving plenary integration; the second step, which should follow naturally from the development of the EIA, is the establishment of enterprise-wide standards. Unfortunately this step depends on the industry as well as the enterprise. Without widely accepted industry standards, an enterprise can become integrated only internally, which is not complete enough.

The task of integration architecture is to define which of these seven levels of integration is needed to support the key business processes. It also must define the details of how and what will be integrated between systems. The decision of which type of integration will be used will have a significant impact on the technology architecture.

Knowledge Architecture

Increasingly, productivity of knowledge will be decisive in its economic and social success, and in its entire economic performance.
—Peter F. Drucker (1993)

In his book *Post-Capitalist Society* (1993), Peter Drucker predicts that knowledge, not capital, will be the primary means of wealth in the 21st century. The current healthcare industry provides an excellent example of his theory. *The heavy dependence on knowledge workers in health care makes the knowledge architecture an essential part of the enterprise information architecture.*

Two of the primary knowledge workers in health care are physicians and nurses. Notes are one tool used to monitor a patient's progress while in the hospital. Since physician and nursing notes are maintained in a free-form text format that is separate from the data they used to make their decisions, this free-form text is much too varied in format for computers to analyze. The knowledge architecture provides a solution. It pinpoints these sources of knowledge, identifies the knowledge workers involved in producing it, and maps both to the enterprise's key business and information processes.

Benefits of an EIA

The primary benefit of an enterprise information architecture is obvious: with a strong EIA in place, an enterprise can more readily ensure changing business processes are being supported by information systems.

However, an enterprise cannot overlook the other direct and indirect benefits of EIA implementation. Used correctly, an architectural approach can:

- Change the focus of IT strategy and planning from a technological and departmental perspective to a business strategy perspective.
- Provide a common and consistent vocabulary and structure that both the IT and business organizations can use to work together.
- Define the business drivers for technology change.
- Complement and enhance the business and strategic planning process.
- Allow changes to either IT or the business to be modeled on paper before implementing.
- Document the complexities of the IT system, allowing new management, employees, and consultants to more quickly understand how both the business and IT work.
- Increase management's confidence that IT is aligned to the business.

Fostering Successful EIA Projects

Unfortunately, the vast majority of EIA projects are not successful. The reasons for failure are classic: lack of support at the executive level, wrong project leaders, lack of methodology, inadequate education on the methodology, and too broad a scope. Enterprises, however, must not stop revising their approaches to EIA implementation. If information management is going to support the growing and varied demands of the enterprise, it must develop an enterprise-wide business process view. The EIA is the first and most important step in achieving this mandate.

The book *Hope Is Not a Method* (Sullivan and Harper 1996) listed rules that led to the successful transformation of their organization. If followed, these rules can also produce a successful EIA:

- Change is hard work.
- Leadership begins with values.
- Expect to be surprised.
- Focus on the future.
- Learn from doing.

The organization that Generals Sullivan and Harper transformed was the U.S. Army. If enterprises follow this code and are unafraid to fail and try again, the EIA will help transform both the IT and business organization.

References

Drucker, P. F. 1993. *Post-Capitalist Society.* New York: Harper Business.

Hewlett Packard/Healthcare Information Management and System Society. 1997. *Annual Leadership Survey.* Chicago: HIMSS.

Inmon, W. 1997. *Data Stores and Data Warehousing and the Zachman Framework.* New York: McGraw-Hill.

Keen, P. 1991. *Shaping the Future: Business Design Through Information Technology.* Boston: Harvard Business School Press.

Sullivan, G. R. and M. V. Harper. 1996. *Hope Is Not a Method: Leadership Lessons for Business from the Transformation of America's Army.* New York: Times Books.

Zachman, J. 1987. "A Framework for Informations Systems Architecture." *IBM Systems Journal* 24(3).

6

Process Design

David Beaulieu

One of the most rewarding endeavors an executive can undertake is sponsoring a successful reengineering effort that improves operational performance to meet strategic business objectives. On the other hand, one of the worst endeavors to undertake is sponsoring a poorly conceived reengineering effort. Despite some well-documented successes associated with "reengineering," "redesign," or "transformation" efforts, most fail miserably and thrust organizations into a deeper level of chaos, resulting in competitive setbacks. We believe the success or failure of reengineering efforts is not a mystery. The outcome is tied directly to the executive's ability to lead, plan, and effectively manage business change by whatever name.

There are many reasons for embarking on major change efforts. Change can, for instance, bail out an organization in decline or help a thriving organization cling to a market-dominant position. However, most executives are concerned with the middle of that spectrum. For them, change is a way to improve overall operational performance and thereby meet enterprise-wide economic, social, and service goals.

The "new think" requires executives to look beyond the barriers imposed by traditional hierarchical and functional organizations and take both vertical and horizontal looks at operational performance. This requires executives to become familiar with process thinking, or operational performance driven by activities cutting across functional and hierarchical units. We present this chapter as a way to manage this "new think." By offering lessons from practical experience and discussing the requirements for successful redesign and reengineering work, we aim to guide executives through the tricky territory of redesign efforts.

Why Projects Fail

With proper leadership and project execution, the chances of delivering a successful project are much improved. *Most projects fail because of poorly executed project fundamentals or a lack of executive oversight, particularly on larger projects.*

Executive involvement, commitment, and leadership of redesign projects often remain at the conceptual level. Clearly, executives must provide leadership and remain committed and involved. That is their job. Many leadership teams do not, however, put substance behind the concept by requiring *action*. Pledging commitment is not enough. A key to project success is developing a plan biased by executive action.

Before sponsoring a process redesign project, executives must be guided by their organization's business plan when selecting appropriate projects that will help attain the organization's objectives. Once projects are selected, executives must play a central role in properly defining, or scoping, the project. Throughout the project, the executive team needs to communicate accurately and to manage expectations about the project's impact on the organization. Skilled project managers who know how to get things done can be invaluable.

Because project management is both science and art, executives need to understand these "early warning signs" so they can resolve problems before they become unmanageable.

Symptoms of Project Problems

- Late completion of activities/deliverables
- Cost overruns
- Substandard performance
- High turnover in project staff and functional staff
- Multiple functional areas performing the same activities on one project
- Executive commitments conflicting with executive behaviors

Causes of Project Problems

- Lack of executive buy-in to the project
- No functional input to planning phase
- No one leader responsible for total project
- Poor control of design changes and customer changes
- Poor understanding of project manager's job
- No integrated planning and control
- Overcommitment of company resources
- Unrealistic planning and scheduling
- Conflicting priorities

When executives observe these symptoms, it is time to ask the right questions to determine if project problems exist. Ignoring these symptoms is the worst thing to do. By taking quick action to remedy the situation, executives can get the team back on track.

Project Planning

The team will be less likely to veer off track if problem prevention starts in the earliest phases of project development. Project planning begins with clear articulation of all players' roles and responsibilities. This requires several planning sessions held between the executive sponsor(s) and project and operations managers. Table 6.1 is a partial sample of how to document who will play what role in a project.

Care should be taken to identify both decision makers and those responsible for *consulting* with stakeholders prior to making the decision and effectively *informing* people about decisions.

Once these roles and responsibilities are established, all those associated with the project must behave accordingly. Executives who have delegated some measure of decision making to subordinates must refrain from "swooping" in and out of the project, indiscriminately making ad hoc decisions that impact progress. If conflicts arise and changes in roles and responsibilities are required, all people involved should be part of that discussion. Eliminating confusion over who does what during various stages of a project can save time, lower project costs, and minimize frustration.

TABLE 6.1. Project roles and responsibilities.

	Project task	Project team	Operation managers	Steering committee	Executive team
Establish organization vision & mission	I	I	C	C	D
Establish organizational goals	I	I	C	C	D
Establish organization budget	I	I	C	C	D
Commission projects	I	I	C	C	D
Establish project ownership	I	I	C	C	D
Establish project governance model & decision making process	I	C	I	C	D
Prioritize projects	I	I	C	C	D
Plan the project	I	D	C	C	C
Set project deadlines & budget	I	C	I	C	D
Establish issues resolution, change control processes	C	D	I	C	C
Complete business case, cost benefit work/return on investment	C	C	D	C	C
Select project manager	I	I	C	C	D
Select team members	I	D	C	C	I
Provide subject matter expertise to team	I	C	D	C	I
Plan communications	I	D	C	C	C
Deliver communications	I	C	C	C	D

Key: D = Decision; C = Consult; I = Inform
© First Consulting Group 1998.

To ensure project success, executives can also:

- Communicate progress regarding change efforts through board meetings, town halls, staff meetings, and public speaking engagements.
- Focus on high-priority projects, with the courage to halt progress on nonessential projects.
- Assist in selecting an experienced project manager and in making personnel changes as different skills are required.
- Build an environment where people can tell the truth and be rewarded for it.
- Understand what is slowing down progress and actively assist in resolving critical issues, removing organizational barriers, and managing conflicting priorities.
- Act as the primary educator of the executive team to gain full consensus for projects.

A key to executive success is the quality and frequency of communications. Successful transformation efforts can be explained quickly and easily, without undue complexity. Communications must be reduced to a few simple messages that executives can present consistently in varied settings.

Another important aspect of communications is clarity of intent. In our experience, most operations people are ready to run—in the opposite direction—at the mention of the word "reengineering." Although "reinventing," "reengineering," and "transforming" have had their evangelists, many operations managers have concluded this is simply another disguise for head count elimination strategies. Get the message straight. Call cost cutting what it is. *Honesty can help improve the organization, even when colleagues know staff will be reduced to eliminate cost.*

Before embarking on a project, discuss and document its financial requirements in full. This is especially important for projects that cross annual budget cycles. Multiyear cross-functional projects cannot be considered part of the typical budget planning process for operations. Invariably, cross-functional infighting will result. At best, this will cause a distraction for the project team. At worst, key project team members will begin to jump ship, as their fate is subject to the budget planning cycle.

The Business Plan

A prerequisite to any major redesign project is a business plan that identifies opportunities for business operational and financial improvement. Redesign efforts that begin before a business plan is developed lack the context needed to rally executive commitment. If they get past the design stage, they generally lose support during implementation and fail to move into production.

Executives may be reluctant to tackle a business planning process because of past disappointments—extended meetings and delays in gaining consensus. We contend, however, that developing a basic business plan need not be a prolonged effort. The outcome should be documentation and communication of the *few* key objectives the project will target over the middle to long term. Once a business plan is developed, all short-term initiatives should be tied to achieving the overarching business objectives. Initiatives that cannot be linked to the business strategy should be eliminated.

A basic business plan must identify the following:

- Customers and suppliers
- Competitors and their strategies
- Products and/or services that meet customers' needs
- Product and/or service performance requirements
- Core processes that deliver the products and/or services
- Enabling information technologies
- Financial requirements.

With a sound business plan in place, the executive has the tools to evaluate how well goals are being met and which areas need improvement.

After problem areas are pinpointed, small assessment teams should assume the responsibility of identifying the root(s) of the performance shortfalls. Traditional views must be challenged by getting to the facts. Assessment teams should avoid the bias to act before understanding the problem, since running to implement preconceived solutions without first identifying the problem will waste time and money. We do not suggest setting immutable deadlines for project completion until a project team is formed and a detailed plan assembled.

Sustainable operational improvement must focus on changing *process* performance. In order to know which processes to work on, it is important to understand which processes drive the appropriate business results. For example, undertaking a massive effort to improve customer relationships by reengineering a customer service/call center might be appropriate if the desired operational improvement is directly or indirectly linked to call center processes. If, however, the key customer dissatisfaction with the organization's performance is untimely and inaccurate delivery of member identification cards, reengineering call centers would not have a measurable impact on the problem. Unfortunately, improving the capabilities of the call center staff might actually mask this problem, since staff will effectively respond to complaints and very few problems will beg for attention.

All this leads to the importance of measuring performance prior to, during, and following all redesign efforts. Measuring process performance during the change effort will make certain executives understand the reason for performance slippage and/or improvement; it will also ensure that the ground gained after implementation is held. This allows the executive team to set new objectives, or "raise the bar"—provided these new performance expectations are clearly articulated.

Process design must support the overarching business objectives of the organization. To make sure this is the case, executives should request a review of the team's business plan *prior* to investing heavily in the redesign process. The objective of a business plan must be kept in mind; ideally, it should document the linkage between a business strategy and the changes in business processes, information technology, and organizations that are planned.

Creating a Business Plan

Before creating a plan, the team must identify the vision for the business area and how the particular initiatives relate to the vision. They should determine competitive position as related to the projects and pinpoint any alternative business scenarios requiring evaluation. Once this is done, they can focus on developing initiatives.

The relationship between the projected initiatives and the likely benefits must be predicted and monitored. After the team outlines the project's functionality, attributes, and revised processes, they should identify benchmarks associated with those revisions. Successful projects require a conceptual framework for calculating benefits levels, a framework including measurement devices that transcend environmental changes. Along the way, accountable operating executives should review the assessment of likely benefits and provide input on the calculation framework.

If the calculation framework is to be of any use, the team must know how to collect data and quantify results. They must request current financial and operating data and consult experts on general financial assumptions concerning tax rates, amortization rules, severance policies, discount rates, capitalization rules, and investment funding.

After implementing the initiatives, the team can quantify benefits by:

- developing a rough frame of reference for the base case view
- determining if benefits are one-time or ongoing
- identifying and quantifying incremental costs associated with achieving benefits
- separating cash flow items from income statement benefits
- calculating profit, cash flow, and investment return.

All this should be completed within a determined project implementation schedule, with a list of nonquantifiable benefits and assumptions close at hand. Teams should also create a management package to accompany the project, complete with a detailed document to be delivered at an executive presentation.

Choosing the Best Approach

There are specific market events that strongly suggest process redesign would be a helpful tool in improving a business. Events that change market conditions and a business's position may include:

- mergers, acquisitions, and divestitures

- consolidations
- new market entries
- departures from a market
- introduction of new competitors in a market
- economic losses (stock position, valuation, etc.)
- leadership changes
- requests for new systems.

Each of these may prompt executives to consolidate business units, adapt best practices for processes, migrate to new technology standards, and revise job classifications and training requirements. Regardless of the event, however, improvement can be attained by managing the complexities of simplifying processes, aligning technology to support new process capabilities, and addressing the requirements of the organization's work force. Incremental gains can be made by attempting to solve a business problem by tackling only one of these areas, but the efforts are usually short-lived.

All components of the change process need to be considered before a project can succeed. That means those process, information technology, and human resource knowledge experts must be part of redesign teams from the outset; if they are not, unnecessary setbacks and delays may result. *We believe working in collaborative teams ensures the best design and the best technology application.* An added benefit is reduced time dedicated to training new team members.

Many new initiatives have been implemented by a healthcare organization's information technology (IT) department without appropriate business sponsorship. In their support, IT executives have been trying to respond to growing business demands to improve customer service and lower operating costs. Information technology has been viewed as a "silver bullet" by many business executives; unfortunately, pure IT efforts to fix service issues and reduce costs have been largely unsuccessful. According to a Gartner Group study, "less than 50 percent of the potential return [of IT investments] flow through the enterprise—inappropriate management practices and work organization for the deployed IT absorbs the balance" (Gartner Group 1996).

Work to change business processes has many names, ranging from "business process reengineering" to "process redesign" to "continuous improvement." Each approach has its appropriate use, depending on the situation. Many examples have been cited in the press regarding the need for radical reengineering, particularly when businesses are failing miserably. Additionally, examples have been presented extolling the ability of total quality management/continuous quality improvement (CQI) to hold gains achieved in the marketplace. Most healthcare organizations neither require radical reengineering nor desire the slower, incremental approach of CQI.

Choosing the right approach depends on the organization's goals and the degree of improvement sought over a predefined time frame. The key factors to consider are the degree of need for change, the pace at which the organization must move, and the amount of risk the organization can tolerate. All this should be clearly articulated in the business plan, and discussion about what is prompting the change should occur at the executive level. There are many possible cases for action: a "near-death" experience, market repositioning for growth, desire to maintain current market position, or the simple fact that "everyone else is doing it." Clearly, executives should be wary of the last option; they should avoid doing anything because it happens to be the latest fad.

Each reasonable case for action has a corresponding approach. A "near-death experience" requires radical reengineering. A drive to dominate the market requires aggressive process redesign. If the organization wishes to simply maintain its current market position, it should espouse CQI. As Figure 6.1 illustrates, however, each approach carries a certain amount of risk.

In general, healthcare organizations have invested significant resources to change processes, introduce enabling technologies, and realign organizations. *The key to success in any business is to recognize what completed work is reusable in the future and what needs to be replaced.* It is probably not acceptable to start from scratch and take a pure reengineering approach, nor is it generally acceptable to take the next decade contemplating the next move. We contend that most organizations would benefit most from a process redesign approach to change.

Executives are becoming familiar with object-oriented design in information technology. The same basic principle—that "modules" of replaceable and interconnected components can be designed—can be applied to both organizational and business process design. This allows executives to plan for significant long-term business change and see progress over the short to middle term by installing "modules" of improvement.

A typical example would be identification of a performance problem in meeting customer service requirements. Many organizations track customer satisfaction through periodic customer service surveys. Once the problem is clearly identified, an assessment team might discover that information to respond to many customer issues is not available to the customer service representatives. Further research also indicates that even if the information were available to customer

Reengineering	Process redesign	Continuous quality improvement (CQI)
High risk, blank piece of paper, dedicated teams, harder to implement, changes process, IT, organization, may not be able to migrate existing business to new environment, capital-intensive, high payoff	Moderate risk, teams integrated with operations, starts with understanding of current performance, gaps, what works already, implementation moderate to difficult depending on scope, impact to process, IT & organization, capital-intensive, high payoff	Low-risk, driven from operations, probably small scope, process only focus, incremental improvements, nonthreatening, small capital requirement, low payoff

FIGURE 6.1 Risks associated with approaches to change
© First Consulting Group 1998.

service representatives, it would be full of inaccuracies. The assessment team then presents a report to the executive team recommending that several expensive and long-term projects be initiated to address the problem. The executive team evaluates the disruption to the organization, the impact of the work on budgets, and the ability to find the right people with knowledge to do the job.

A modular approach to improving customer satisfaction might be to design changes in enrollment/eligibility, changing contract documentation, upgrading the desktop, automating benefit descriptions, and so forth. Each might contribute in a smaller way to enhancing customer satisfaction in the middle term through delivery of improvements every three to six months, even though the full project might take three years.

To begin design work, a team must identify basic design principles that will act as the foundation for their work. Basic design principles must be reviewed with the executive team and sign-off obtained. Design principle examples include:

- designing new processes with the fewest possible steps
- collecting information once
- collecting information as close to the source as possible
- storing information in one place
- designing processes for greatest customer satisfaction
- designing for the lowest possible costs
- designing for elimination of cycle time.

In addition to design principles, the team must identify the critical success factors necessary to ensure success. These might include:

- establishing a governance committee
- obtaining executive commitment
- obtaining appropriate and sustained funding
- selecting the right project manager and team
- obtaining the support from key operations managers
- constructing a solid project plan
- establishing end-user review teams.

An important objective of the executive team is to identify behaviors that have led to project success and failure in the organization's past. With this understanding, executives should lead the team to repeat the successful behaviors. Likewise, executives must be attentive when members of their organizations repeat behaviors that have led to project failure. Obviously, stopping ineffective behavior—particularly at the executive level—is one of the most critical necessities in a redesign effort.

There are many different methodologies on the market today. Though many people attempt to sell executives on why their method is the time-proven best, it is important to remember that all competent methodologies are basically the same. The key differentiator is in *how* a sound methodology is used. A methodology is only a means to a desired end; if it does not help to successfully design or implement solutions, then it should not be used. Likewise, if certain steps in a methodology do not help move the organization to the desired goal, then they should be skipped. Methodologies are best used as guidebooks for experienced process designers. They should assist smart people in completing the redesign work, in implementing new processes, and in introducing enabling technology.

Measurement

In order to reach new levels of operational performance, it is critical that business processes be measured. Each process must generate specific measurable outcomes. These include quality, service, cost, and cycle time performance.

As discussed earlier, it is crucial to assess the outcomes produced by current processes. These results should be compared to the goals set for the organization by the executive team. A gap analysis should then be completed to document the improvement needed to meet the organization's business objectives.

A detailed discussion of measurable performance improvement should be included in the business case. Ultimately, this work will be fine-tuned to generate a cost/benefit analysis, including return on investment (ROI) calculations. It is important to measure *business operations performance;* avoid doing cost/benefit and ROI calculations on information technology investments. As John Glasser points out,

> . . . information systems have no value outside of the organization's strategies and plans: They must arise from and support these strategies and plans. For example, if we intend to improve the quality of our care, what information system capabilities and related investments are necessary? (Glaser 1997, p. 134)

Measurement of an organization's process capabilities can take several forms. At the macro level, a measurement capability should be established to provide the executive team with critical information on how well the organization is performing against key strategic objectives. This "executive dashboard" should be limited to the truly important items that executives use to make decisions. An example of an executive dashboard is illustrated in Table 6.2.

An executive dashboard can be developed by following a few simple steps:

- Identify key measurements impacting business (financial results, growth, customer and supplier satisfaction, employee satisfaction).
- Identify reporting formats, frequency, and audiences.
- Identify reporting process and accountabilities.
- Identify IT enablers.

From a project redesign standpoint, measurements should also be put in place to track progress. This includes use of a project management tool like reporting

TABLE 6.2. Sample health plan "executive dashboard."

Critical performance indicator	Measurement: Financial/cost	Quality	Service	Time
Profitability	• >5% return on equity • MLR <84%			
Customer service	• Administrative cost ratio <11% • 100% premium bills accurate	• Claim payments 98% + accurate • ID cards correct • <1% member grievances/year • 100% call center responses accurate • 100% buyer reports accurate	• 90% + top 2/5 in survey • 80% calls answered in 20 seconds	• 100% members receive ID cards prior to effective date • 100% buyers receive bills 1st of month
Provider service	• Cost/claim under $2.50	• 99.8% financial accuracy claim payments • 100% capitation accuracy • <3% capitation adjustments	• 90% + top 2/5 in survey • < 5% referral complaints	• 100% capitation paid on 15th of month
Employee satisfaction	• <10% turnover	• 100% salary actions accurate	• 95% + top 2/5 in survey	• 100% employees have job objectives • 100% appraisals on time

© First Consulting Group 1998.

against key milestones. In addition, large projects should be supported with an issues tracking, escalation, and resolution process.

Focus, Impatience, and Perseverance

The most difficult phase of a redesign project is neither the kickoff nor the implementation. The executive team and the organization in general share a high level of enthusiasm as a new project is kicked off. Everyone is involved, communications are frequent, and executives are highly visible. A similar level of interest and enthusiasm is present during implementations, with particular involvement from operations leaders and their staffs.

One of the most difficult executive tasks is continued focus and attention to projects as they go beyond kickoff stages into detailed design, construction of solutions, testing, and preparation for implementation. Much work is happening behind the scenes without much apparent payoff. Now is the time to reenergize executive involvement, directing it at the needs of the project manager and team.

Progress discussions are more crucial now than ever; they should continue in regular executive sessions. The executive team should help others in the organization maintain their focus on meeting the needs of the project, including continued access to subject matter experts, the reabsorption of project team members into operations, and the use of operations staff to complete reviews and sign-off of new process designs, particularly in preparation for acceptance testing and implementation.

At all stages of redesign projects, executives should be looking for opportunities to implement modules of new process design. The ability to establish early victories for the organization is important to the project team's credibility. If done properly, this also gives executives a measure of early success in the life cycle of a larger project. This can be important in preparing updates for board presentations, in justifying project funding, and in demonstrating to managers the value of the redesign team's contributions to operations.

Before kicking off a new project, executives should form an assessment team to sketch out a high-level project plan. This will help clarify the complexities of a larger project and define the actual work that needs to be done to create a series of deliverables. An unhealthy tension usually develops between project and executive teams when executives set target delivery dates in the absence of a detailed plan. This can immediately put the project manager at extremely high risk for not delivering in alignment with executive expectations. In the worst situations, project teams compromise the deliverable by changing scope or cutting corners to deliver some capability on time. Executive patience is key to completing an effective planning effort so decision makers understand the magnitude of investment required to deliver new business processes, technology, and organizational designs.

Once a project plan has been developed and delivery dates identified, it is important for executives to demonstrate *impatience* throughout the life of the project. The focus must be on generating results. Executive impatience will help the project team quickly remove barriers hindering team progress.

Embarking on large-scale redesign efforts takes courage. Organizations attempting such efforts are often attacked by critics full of reasons why the effort should be discontinued. Still, as long as project management discipline is in place, the right people are doing the work, and strong leaders are present and committed, perseverance will conquer most obstacles. *Executives must remember that people gravitate toward the familiar; the challenge is learning how to pull them to the future.*

Managing Risk and Pace

Large-scale projects should be broken down into a number of smaller, manageable projects. Although substantial operational improvement can be realized during the long-term project, incremental improvement should be demonstrated throughout the life of large-scale redesign projects. Key milestones should be established to demonstrate short-term successes. We suggest a key deliverable be planned every three to six months and reviewed with the executive team.

Project risk can be minimized by following some basic guidelines in developing projects plans:

- Projects must be directly tied to the organization's business plan.
- Projects must deliver measurable operational improvement.
- Projects must be carefully planned, deliverables must be clearly defined, and timetables must be driven from these plans, not from arbitrary executive decisions.
- Projects should have periodic milestones in which incremental operational improvements are implemented.
- Projects must have the sustained commitment of an executive team that is communicating enthusiasm to the rest of the organization over the entire project.
- Projects must focus on design of business processes to deliver sustainable operational improvement.
- Processes should be designed, enabling technology delivered, and organization alignment completed to support the organization's business objectives.
- All improvements should be implemented by operations people, who must be involved in all phases of the project (including design sessions, testing, and implementation).
- Appropriate levels of financial and subject matter resources must be provided to deliver project results.
- The organization's work must focus on a few critical projects and reject additional requests that would create constraints.

Above all, executives must remember that *process redesign is not a spectator sport*. Everyone on the team must actively participate in the game on the field. Be wary of people who want to be spectators; find out why they are reluctant to participate, then get them actively involved. Do not neglect the role of the human resource staff: engage them in developing and taking leadership responsibility for communications planning, training development, scheduling, rewriting job descriptions, evaluating performance management capabilities, and addressing compensation requirements.

During executive sessions, routinely discuss the pace of projects and the risks to the organization and the project team. With the project manager, actively evaluate progress against plans. Remove barriers. Constantly solicit help and demand executive support for the change effort. Know when to be a team member and when to be a leader.

After investing heavily in a redesign project, it is important to preserve the gains attributed to implementation. On an organization-wide basis, how is success measured? We believe the key is to track performance before, during, and after the implementation of new processes, IT, and organizational capabilities. Ask this question of staff members: "As a result of this change effort, what are you doing differently on Monday morning at the start of your work day?" If they cannot answer that simple question, successes can never be sustained because nothing has truly changed.

Done properly, redesign efforts do substantially boost an organization's ability to deliver improved, sustainable operational performance. Successful projects eliminate unnecessary delays, improve customer service and quality, and reduce costs. Focusing on project management basics, communicating clearly and consistently, and delivering superior leadership over the course of redesign projects will not only help an organization achieve the goals articulated in the business plan, they will also make process redesign a very rewarding experience.

References

Gartner Group. 1996. "How Do You Prioritize Investment and Reinvestment?" A Gartner Research Note (EAME), April 8.

Glasser, J. 1997. "Beware Return on Investment." *Healthcare Informatics,* June, 134.

7

Care Delivery and Care Management

Barbara Hoehn and Leslie Perreault

In today's rapidly changing healthcare environment, integrated delivery networks (IDNs) are facing unique challenges in the clinical setting (Coddington et al. 1996). Patient care delivery has expanded outside the four walls of the hospital, coordinated care management is bridging the continuum of care, and efforts to manage costs without jeopardizing quality are paramount in all markets, regardless of managed care market stage (Shortell et al. 1996). Initiatives to vertically integrate multiple clinical entities into a single full-service care provider will present both operational and information integration challenges. Coordinating the management and delivery of patient care services across multiple geographic environments and across time will challenge current processes and information systems. As these trends continue, IDNs must learn to create integrated cross-continuum clinical processes supported by seamless information access, communication, and management (Coffey et al. 1997).

If IDNs are to implement these strategies successfully, we believe they will need to coordinate clinical services effectively across the care continuum and across traditional clinical disciplines, as well as be clinically efficient and effective within each of the care provider entities of the IDN. The challenge is how to make that happen (FCG 1997).

Clinical initiatives addressing data communication and exchange have historically fallen under the purview of information systems projects. Clinical initiatives addressing care workflow, clinical efficiency, and clinical effectiveness are addressed in clinical redesign or reengineering efforts. All too often these projects are conducted in vacuums with little integration, coordination, or input across project teams. We believe this happens because performance improvement efforts and information management projects have been perceived as solutions to separate problems rather than two components of a single problem's solution. Furthermore, while individual healthcare providers have achieved some benefits from both redesign and information systems projects, true clinical transformation and maximum benefits achievement will not be realized until an integrated process and information management solution is applied.

The Clinical Informatics Model

Clinical informatics is the integration of newly designed or redesigned clinical processes, information, and information technologies to meet the needs of clinical decision makers (Hoehn and Ball 1997). The clinical informatics model examines clinical processes that are focused on the relationships, activities, and outcomes of the interactions between:

- the patient and direct care provider (patient-focused processes)
- patient populations and clinical evaluators (population-focused processes)
- the members and the care manager (member-focused processes).

The model then identifies the information access, delivery, and management mechanisms needed to support them. These mechanisms are illustrated in Figure 7.1.

Types of Management/Delivery Processes

In the clinical setting, there are three major care management and care delivery processes:

- **Patient-focused clinical processes**—those processes that address the interaction between the clinical care provider and the individual patient or client in providing access to care, delivering episodic care, managing care delivery, and evaluating the patient's outcomes from services provided.

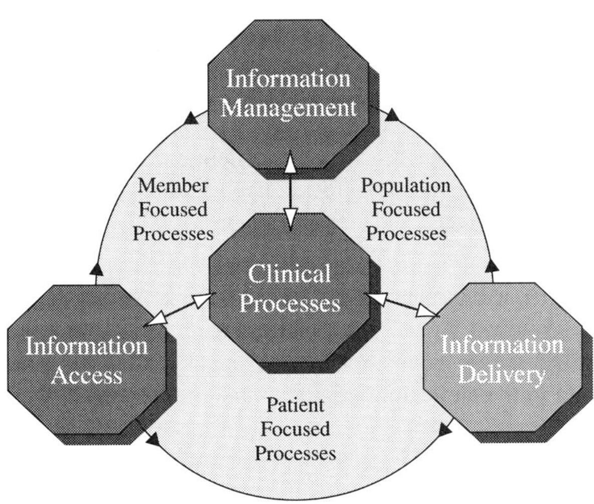

FIGURE 7.1. Clinical Information Delivery Model
© First Consulting Group 1998

- **Population-focused clinical processes**—those processes that address the service delivery needs of specific patient populations (by diagnosis, age, geographic region) and support the clinicians in defining, evaluating, and disseminating best clinical practices.
- **Member-focused clinical processes**—those processes that address the service needs of the covered lives that are the responsibility of the IDS and support the case managers' and clinical administrators' decision-making efforts.

All too often, at least in the traditional information technology approach, we confuse clinical processes with clinical activities and focus on how automation will allow clinicians to perform tasks differently. *When looking at an information management approach, we need to expand our view to include all the components of the clinical process and all the parameters involved.* Each component will have different information implications.

Components of Clinical Processes

There are six major components associated with clinical processes. *Clinical activities* are the tasks and work steps associated with a care process and the facilities, materials, and resource levels needed to perform the activities. *Organizations, roles, and skills* reflect the knowledge, decision-making, and responsibility levels of the professionals involved in the clinical process. *Performance measures* are the matrices used to measure the success of the process and the success of the care provider. (They may be measures of clinical outcomes as well as measures of clinical efficiency.) *Organizational culture* represents the attitudes of teamwork, clinical behavior, and styles and the impact of these attitudes on achieving the clinical objective. The *paradigms* define the change strategies that will activate clinical decisions and achieve successful solutions, and *strategies* reflect how the clinical process supports the objectives of the IDN.

To support these clinical processes, we need to apply information science techniques (data modeling, data structures, data definitions, and linkages) and information technologies (networks, platforms, applications, and resources) to meet the information access, delivery, and management needs of the clinical decision maker.

Integrating Processes and Information

Tables 7.1 to 7.3 reflect the integration of clinical processes and information vehicles inherent in the clinical informatics model.

Examples of Clinical Processes

Using the clinical informatics model of performance improvement through information management, consider an example from each of the clinical process groups: patient-focused, population-focused, and member-focused processes.

TABLE 7.1. Patient-focused processes.

Clinical informatics: Meeting the needs of the patient and care provider			
Patient-focused clinical processes	Information access	Information delivery	Information management
• Identify patient/ member • Schedule encounter/ resource • Register/enroll patient • Verify benefits/ eligibility • Obtain authorization to treat • Manage referrals • Access patient history • Evaluate patient condition • Diagnose • Plan care • Deliver services • Document care • Report results • Manage compliance to care	• Local area and wide area networks (LANs/WANs) • Integration engines • Point-of-care technology • Mobile computing • Remote access • Graphical user interface (GUI) • Clinical informaticians • Unique patient identifier • Smart cards • Patient access/input	• Rules-based orders management • Integrated results • Patient scheduling • Patient management • Clinical ancillary systems • Ambulatory records • Critical care systems • Home care systems	• Document imaging • Longitudinal patient history • Health record • Family record • Integrated data repositories • Specialty databases

© First Consulting Group 1998

Patient-Focused Process: Cross-Continuum Care Management

Centered in primary care, cross-continuum care management is based on principles of population-care management, multidiscipline teamwork, and a network of coordinated clinical services to meet the needs of each patient.

The clinical process of providing, managing, evaluating, and improving care across the continuum consists of the components shown in Table 7.4.

Though the information challenges of cross-continuum care management are daunting, three levels of information management support can help overcome the obstacles. The first level is support to the primary care provider/case manager. Internal electronic mail among members of the care team—including physicians, nurse practitioners, home care providers, and allied health professionals—is an important first tool in facilitating information communication and management. More advanced applications like electronic patient rosters, documentation and variance reporting tools, initial and ongoing patient assessments, and contacts are already available in today's commercial marketplace. If the role of the care provider/care manager is to be fully supported, it will be crucial to expand these systems for broader use across care settings. Integration of these applications

TABLE 7.2. Population-focused processes.

Clinical informatics: Meeting the needs of the population and care evaluator			
Population-focused clinical processes	Information access	Information delivery	Information management
• Develop protocols and guidelines • Monitor quality indicators • Identify and respond to protocol variances • Evaluate resource utilization and costs of care • Assess, evaluate, and track outcomes • Profile providers • Provide clinical education • Expand clinical knowledge bases • Support research • Measure compliance to care	• Networks • Integration engines • Clinical thesaurus • Security plans • Computing cycles • Remote access • Natural language query • Statistical analysis • Internet access	• Clinical libraries • Knowledge databases • Cost accounting • Quality management • Critical paths • E-mail • Bulletin boards • Point-of-care rules-based decision support	• Statistical software • Integrated clinical and financial repositories • Outcomes management • Variance reporting

© First Consulting Group 1998

TABLE 7.3. Member-focused processes.

Clinical informatics: Meeting the needs of the member and care manager			
Member-focused clinical processes	Information access	Information delivery	Information management
• Assign clinical • Collect and archive clinical data • Coordinate hand-offs between providers • Monitor compliance to care • Identify and monitor at-risk populations • Manage risks and liabilities	• Networks • Integration engines • Clinical dictionaries • Case managers • Ad hoc queries	• Case management • Variance reporting • Protocol libraries • Rules-based clinical systems • Integrated scheduling • Referral management systems • Cost accounting applications • Decision support	• Longitudinal patient histories • Case mix data • Patient/member profiles • Profit/loss information • Disease management

© First Consulting Group 1998

TABLE 7.4. Cross-continuum care management model.

Strategy	Cross-continuum care	Both the patient and the care system will achieve benefits through coordination and continuity of patient management provided in the most appropriate setting
Paradigm	Population-based management	Care will be based upon best practices developed through the analysis of care delivered to populations of patients characterized as subgroups with distinct medical and psychosocial characteristics
Clinical activities	Care models	Care models will be developed and/or adapted to meet the needs of patient populations, addressing how care is accessed and delivered and what care is delivered
Organization, roles, and skills	Teamwork	Care management includes the coordinated interplay of a set of competencies and integrating primary and specialty care in a unified approach. Also includes extended care team of home providers
Culture	Personal health management	Patients will be guided or coached to adopt best practices in personal health management. Providers will be assisted in consistently doing the right thing for their patients
Performance measures	Protocols	Clinical guidelines and protocols based on demonstrated epidemiological evidence will drive care delivery

© First Consulting Group 1998

with patient and resource scheduling, core and advanced clinical functionality, and longitudinal patient data will also be paramount.

The second level of information management support deals with care sites involved in cross-continuum patient management programs. Most cross-continuum care management programs are initially focused on high-risk patients for whom special practices or clinics are established. These clinics are involved in screening and intake functions as well as patient management activities. Data access and communication can be supported by the most robust of current ambulatory systems; however, screening and care management functions are still generally unsupported, and true protocol-based care management will not be supported until the ambulatory patient management and documentation systems can support pathway algorithms, variance monitoring, and rules-based decision support at the point of care.

The third level is enterprise-wide support in the health system. Patient tracking, patient care assignments, and real-time information on the primary care team must be maintained for all patients within the health system. The ability to support outcomes analysis and program management will be a crucial factor in successfully implementing and conducting a cross-continuum care management program. Here, too, patient-specific clinical decision support systems are important in ensuring that the care team follows through with planned interventions and is alerted early to unplanned events that could affect clinical outcomes.

Population-Focused Process: Adopting Best Practices

As IDNs take on responsibility for the health status of defined populations, they are increasingly concerned with measuring and managing variations in care delivery practices, clinical outcomes, and costs of care. Identifying and adopting clinical best practices entails ongoing evaluation of care delivery practices and outcomes; it also means that mechanisms to influence provider behavior must be implemented.

Table 7.5 illustrates the process of measuring clinical outcomes and managing to best practices.

As managed care leads physicians and administrators toward a common goal of providing high-quality yet cost-effective health care, there is an increasing emphasis within IDNs on identifying and implementing best practices. With appropriate physician leadership and participation, we believe that focusing on best

TABLE 7.5. Best practices model.

Strategy	Identification and adoption of best practices	Both the patient and the care system will benefit from evaluation of care delivery practices and adoption of current best practices by all providers
Paradigm	Population-based management	Care will be based upon best practices developed through the analysis of care delivered to population of patients characterized as subgroups with distinct medical and psychosocial characteristics
Clinical activities	Evidence-based medicine	Providers will practice in accordance with institutionally determined standards of care designed to improve clinical outcomes, reduce costs, and minimize unexplained variability
Organization, roles, and skills	Physician and administrative collaboration	Development of practice standards extends quality improvement initiatives to clinical processes; physicians and administration will collaborate in evaluation of current practices and clinical quality improvement
Culture	Explicit practice guidelines	Deployment of best practices requires that clinicians alter their practice behaviors in response to evidence of more effective approaches to patient care
Performance measures	Clinical outcomes management	Provider performance will be evaluated relative to current best practices to identify and incorporate better approaches, educate individual practitioners, and cultivate agreement among providers

© First Consulting Group 1998

practices provides an excellent opportunity to improve clinical outcomes and reduce clinical practice variation, thereby reducing costs.

Besides addressing technological issues, an IDN must focus on organizational issues to ensure measurable performance improvement. Challenges include developing organizational structures that encourage physicians to work together, implementing shared financial incentives (e.g., capitated payments for physician services), and managing perceived legal concerns (e.g., possible malpractice risk due to deviation from clinical guidelines).

Clinical information systems support plays a major role in both the development and implementation of clinical best practices. The systems are crucial, for instance, in the development of clinical guidelines. A consensus approach to developing clinical guidelines is often an IDN's first step toward adopting institution-specific standards of care. Evaluating patient clinical data across population subgroups can assist in guidelines development by providing objective evidence of variance in services and outcomes. Once developed, these guidelines can be refined through the use of clinical information systems that document interventions and clinical outcomes. Developing ambulatory patient information systems will be critical to the capture of clinical information in physician office settings.

Data used to develop guidelines are relatively easy to gather; for instance, claims data for inpatient and outpatient encounters are widely available and can be supplemented with clinical data subsets abstracted from patient medical records. Regardless of the sources and extent of the data collected, implementing analytical tools and an integrated database (outcomes database or data warehouse) will be necessary to support iterative analysis of the clinical, financial, and administrative data collected from the various care settings.

To ensure that current best practices for cross-continuum care management are communicated, we believe online access to diagnosis-specific guidelines should be provided. Once they are on the Internet, these guidelines can serve as references for clinicians caring for patients with selected chronic diseases or high-cost conditions. Retrospective analysis of variations in clinical practices and outcomes (for example, through comparative provider profiles) offers another basic means for evaluating and altering clinician behavior. These systems will integrate online clinical documentation, assessment, planning, and ordering functions with point-of-care decision-support tools, including alerts, reminders, and real-time variance management. *Patient-specific information on best practices must be available to clinicians at the place and time clinical decisions are made* if IDNs are to maximize their impact on clinician practice patterns.

Member-Focused Process: Referrals Management

Referrals management in the traditional sense entails determination by providers of a member's eligibility for referral services, depending on payer rules and member history. Narrowly defined as such, referrals management can be equated with referral authorization. As IDNs increasingly assume risk for the cost and outcomes of care provided, they have both a greater opportunity and a greater need to internalize the referrals management function—to manage referrals according to their own assessment of clinical appropriateness, with consideration for customer service requirements. An IDN's ability to take advantage of this increased control will depend on the organization's capacity for cross-continuum care management according to best practices and principles of evidence-based medicine.

The process of referrals management consists of the components shown in Table 7.6. Eventually, any provider strategy that aims to manage costs and quality through cross-continuum care management will be led by medical necessity rather than payer rules when investing in policies, procedures, and systems for referrals management. In an environment of local competition, an IDN may provide a user-friendly referral management process to encourage regional providers to do business with them. More advanced organizations may selectively assume risk where they believe they can manage a process more efficiently internally. For IDNs with a health plan component, referrals management can reduce costs and improve member satisfaction by optimizing the efficiency of the referral process—getting the patient appointed with the correct generalist or specialist at the first encounter.

TABLE 7.6. Referrals management model.

Strategy	Referrals management	Both the patient and IDN will benefit from the management of referrals according to IDN-determined assessments of clinical and/or service appropriateness
Paradigm	Member-based management	Clinical appropriateness will be determined through analysis of care delivered and customer service requirements of patient and member subpopulations with distinct medical and psychosocial characteristics
Clinical activities	Medical management	Providers will refer for specialty services in accordance with institutionally determined standards of care designed to improve clinical outcomes, reduce costs, minimize unexplained variances, and maintain customer satisfaction
Organization, roles, and skills	Physician integration	Physicians and medical administration will define and adopt rules for determining what referral services are clinically appropriate, when authorizations are needed, and where referral services can be provided
Culture	Risk sharing	Physicians and IDN cooperate in managing risk by standardizing care through implementation of referral rules and practice guidelines
Performance measures	Risk management	The IDN effectively manages risk by controlling utilization of specialty services and out-of-network referrals

© First Consulting Group 1998

The referral process is one that bridges traditional boundaries of care, entering into the realm of cross-continuum care management. We believe the ability to manage and control such cross-continuum processes will be essential to the success of any IDN, particularly if its leaders are risk takers. In the short term, however, few organizations—other than those in which all providers are owned or employed—are in a position to manage the combined information systems and provider relations challenges necessary to accomplish this goal.

Critical organizational success factors include tight integration of physicians into the organizational structures and operations of the IDN. For example, provider integration within a medical service organization (MSO) with significant contracting power is advantageous—the MSO will have substantial leverage with their providers and payors, thus providing the basis for coordinated initiatives to standardize care by implementing practice guidelines and protocols. Without significant physician integration, referrals management is likely to remain the more traditional referral authorization. A major operational challenge is obtaining consistent referral rules from medical administration—specifically, learning from the administration precisely how they wanted the rules to operate. The more complex the organization for medical management, the greater the task of explicating the different medical management rules and contact terms.

The extent of an IDN's ability to manage referrals is heavily dependent on the organization's information management infrastructure. A successful infrastructure should fulfill two main requirements: it should provide ample communication and guidance, and it should integrate referral rules into the process of care.

Communication and Guidance

At the least sophisticated end of the information systems spectrum, physician practices may have at their disposal only telephone, fax, and mail as means of communicating referral information. Electronic mail—provided by the IDN or purchased independently by providers—provides a next level of connectivity, enabling rapid exchange of referral requests, and even scheduling of referral services, without requiring simultaneous connectivity between parties. However, we need to incorporate more sophisticated mechanisms for guiding the referrals process if we are to move beyond simple referral authorization to policy-driven referrals management.

Implementation of Internet and intranet technologies holds promise in delivery of system applications to end users; for example, development of a web-browser interface to an IDN's managed care system can allow provider offices to obtain real-time approval or denial of referrals based on referral rules embedded in the system's logic. Online referral forms can prompt requests for valid reasons for the referral and offer a checklist of approved referral service providers. Electronic messaging, with appropriate security, can allow communication between referring and consulting physicians; the referring physician can append clinical summary data and notes, and the consultant can give electronic feedback on her findings. In this way, the system can facilitate both medical management and the authorization of referrals.

Integrating Referral Rules

We have no doubt that expanded functionality and tight linkages with scheduling, registration, and clinical systems are necessary to truly manage the referral process. If an organization is to develop and deploy its own standards and referral rules for clinical appropriateness, then it requires underlying access to clinical, financial, and administrative data from physician offices and other care settings. Incorporating referrals management into call center operations or other access care processes affords the opportunity for direct referral to a specialist by a triage nurse according to complaint-specific clinical protocols.

Integral to this approach is access to core clinical systems, a capability that allows triage nurses to view patient clinical data at the time of the call. Similarly, embedding referrals management within care delivery systems and processes minimizes redundant data capture and guides clinicians according to explicit practice guidelines. Here, too, point-of-care clinical systems for documentation, assessment, planning, order management, and clinical decision support will enable appropriate use of referral services.

Clinical Informatics: Putting It All Together

Only through an integrated approach—one that accounts for clinical process, organization, and information management—will organizations maximize the benefits of their clinical initiatives. Using the clinical process view, an IDN can assess its organizational and technological strengths and barriers and develop programs that align and coordinate the organization's clinical efforts. A highly sophisticated new care model will remain on the shelf until the IDN has implemented its fundamental information systems infrastructure. Similarly, the promised benefits of enormous investments in sophisticated information technology will remain largely unrealized if physicians do not share in IDN leadership and cooperate in risk management.

Clinical informatics, a process perspective that focuses on patients, members, and population, can help an IDN articulate clear strategies, define measurable performance outcomes, and develop complete programs to implement these strategies successfully. If an IDN is to achieve true clinical transformation, we believe its leaders must begin by adopting this process-oriented perspective on care delivery and care management.

References

Coddington, D.C., K.D. Moore, and E.A. Fischer. 1996. *Making Integrated Health Care Work*. Engelwood, Colo.: Center for Research in Ambulatory Health Care Administration.

Coffey, R.J., Fenner, K.M., and Stogis, S.L. 1997. *Virtually Integrated Health Systems*. San Francisco: Jossey-Bass.

First Consulting Group. 1997. "New Models for Cross-Continuum Care Management: IDN of the 21st Century," *Emerging Practices White Paper,* March. Long Beach, Calif.: FCG.

Hoehn, B.J. and M.J. Ball. 1997. "Clinical Informatics: A Patient-Centric Approach," in *Clinical Information Systems,* Vol. 1, Hospital-Based Systems, eds. M.J. Ball and J.V. Douglas. Redmond, Wash.: SpaceLabs Medical.

Shortell, S.M., R.R Gillies, D.A. Anderson, K.M. Erickson, and J.B. Mitchell. 1996. *Remaking Health Care in America: Building Organized Delivery Systems.* San Francisco: Jossey-Bass.

8

Health Plan Operations and Marketing: The Emerging Network Manager Role

JAMES R. MCPHAIL AND ROBERT G. BONSTEIN, JR.

The growth of managed care in the delivery of health care has placed into motion a dramatic shift in the role of healthcare organizations (HCOs). Health systems that understand this unprecedented change in how health care is delivered *and* are able to adapt to this new environment will obtain the ultimate market advantage. The rewards will belong to those HCOs that can most quickly and successfully adopt the new role of "network manager."

We believe the time is right for HCOs to address this critical issue, since the healthcare cost and access crisis continues to intensify. From 1960 to 1995, national health expenditures in the United States increased from $27.1 billion to $988.5 billion (Health Insurance Association, 1997, p. 99). The Health Care Financing Administration (HCFA) predicts that government expenditures for health care will reach almost $700 billion by the year 2000 (Health Insurance Association 1996, p. 59). Despite these increased expenditures, the percentage of U.S. population without health insurance has been steadily increasing. In 1988, 15.2 percent of the nonelderly population was uninsured, and by 1995, this percentage had increased to 17.4 percent (Mullen 1995).

Healthcare distribution channels are rapidly shifting to various forms of managed care as healthcare purchasers attempt to deal with this ongoing crisis. HCOs must now compete for patients that belong to a variety of prepaid purchasing groups like CHAMPUS, Medicare and Medicaid Risk, and Commercial HMO. A variety of managed care products are becoming associated with these distribution channels as the shift from traditional fee-for-service indemnity continues.

One of the most dramatic shifts in distribution channels is the extremely rapid movement of Medicare and Medicaid populations to prepaid risk plans. A majority of states now have Medicaid risk programs, and large states like California and Texas are shifting their Medicaid populations into managed care risk products in an effort to decrease costs and/or increase population coverage by these programs. Recently, the number of Medicaid participants in managed care programs has been doubling each year.

Medicare managed care growth has also been considerable. In 1996, an average of 80,000 Medicare recipients enrolled in HMOs each month (Health Insurance Association 1996). As of June 1997, there were 283 Medicare risk plans with 4,700,386 enrollees. This encompasses 12.7 percent of all beneficiaries (Health Insurance Association 1997).

Some HCOs may disagree about the transition to managed care and the need for a network manager emphasis. They will argue that the status quo can be maintained forever, especially in secondary markets. Given the lack of managed care penetration in certain parts of the country, this skepticism is understandable. Such skeptics, however, have failed to grasp the rapid growth of managed care (in particular Medicare and Medicaid programs) and the ongoing healthcare cost and access crisis. *No matter what form it takes, managed care is here to stay.*

The Network Manager Role

Although HCOs must continue in their traditional patient care capacity, they must also take on and integrate the network manager functions with the patient care processes. Table 8.1 highlights some of the traditional characteristics of an HCO versus the new roles for the network manager.

As the table indicates, being a network manager is a difficult job. The typical large network manager must:

- manage thousands of physicians, facilities, labs, home health agencies, and other healthcare providers as part of multiple virtual provider contracting networks
- administer a hundred or more separate provider contracts associated with the provider contracts, which have a wide variety of financial terms
- identify and administer properly tens of thousands of customers accessing the various network configurations

TABLE 8.1. Network manager characteristics.

Characteristics	Traditional role	Network manager role
Distribution channels	• Physicians • "Ask a Nurse" call center • Emergency room	• Medicare provider service organization (PSO) • Carve-out product • Medicare risk contracts or product • HMO product • CHAMPUS contract
Key business processes	• Patient accounting • Patient scheduling and registration	• Network administration • Contract administration • Medical management
Core application components	• Scheduling • Registration • Lab • Radiology	• Capitation management • Credentialing • HEDIS reporting • Provider management
Performance metrics	• Inpatient admissions • Bed utilization	• % write-off of managed care contracts • Membership • Medical loss ratio

© First Consulting Group 1998

- administer unique and referral requirements for numerous combinations of payer, employer, network, product, and benefit plan type
- administer and reconcile complex capitation payment rules.

Integrating Managed Care Processes

Besides shouldering responsibility for challenging new tasks, the network manager must gain the support of new business processes. For the network manager business model to come together and deliver health care in the new managed care environment, new managed care business processes must be integrated in five functional areas:

- **Point-of-care support.** Point-of-care support includes all activities that must take place during the patient care process. Key business processes that must be supported in this area include utilization management, demand management, disease management, and referral management. Referral management is of particular importance to determine whom a patient can be referred to within the relevant network and to avoid "network leakage" and the resulting financial losses.
- **Daily operational support.** Network administration is one of the most critical processes associated with operational support. The network manager must be able to build and maintain multiple virtual contracting networks encompassing all aspects of the healthcare delivery equation. Other key processes in this area include claims and encounter administration, customer service, and membership. Membership is a good example of the current inability of health systems to identify the health plan relationship of patients at registration. When a patient walks in the door, a competent network manger must be able to identify that patient's managed care demographics, including membership, primary care physician, benefits, copay, etc.
- **Back office operations.** This area encompasses those processes that support "behind the scenes" functions occurring on a weekly, monthly, or annual basis. Examples of typical managed care processes here would be financial management and quality and outcomes management.
- **Clinical and financial information management.** A lack of good information for managed care decision-making purposes is commonplace with healthcare organizations today. Important processes here for network managers include provider profiling, performance reporting tools like Healthplan Employer Data and Information Set (HEDIS), and various quality measures for patient satisfaction, process, and outcomes.
- **Contract administration.** Health systems currently participate in a wide variety of managed care contracts with various financial terms. Key processes for the network manager in this area are contract management and capitation man-

agement. These processes help the network manager monitor financial performance in the new managed care world. For example, many health systems are entering into very large capitation contracts but have no mechanism in place to track whether these risk contracts are profitable, let alone what the profit margin or loss is. Even for "nonrisk" contracts like discounts or per diems, providers are typically underpaid by five to six percent on contract terms, and they have not yet invested in the necessary processes and systems to ensure appropriate payment—even though these systems can pay for themselves within 12 months!

New Information Technologies

New managed care business processes require new enabling information technology (IT). Many industries invest between 5 and 10 percent of revenues in information technology and commit over 50 percent of annual capital expenditures to IT, a level of investment the healthcare industry does not approach. Most HCOs prefer to spend their capital on "bricks and mortar," operating suites, cath labs, and magnetic resonance imaging, despite the low utilization of these resources in many areas of the country. *To operate more efficiently, HCOs must begin to embrace the substitution of fixed cost information technology for variable cost labor.*

The following are some samples of application components:

- **Claims and encounter administration.** Key application components under this crucial process include claims and encounter adjudication, claims audit, benefits administration, and other claims modules such as dental, pharmacy, and vision. These application components are necessary to support the collection of encounter data in tracking the performance of risk contracts by the network manager.
- **Capitation management.** Application components here include capitation administration, underwriting, and actuarial and premium billing. This is where capitation contract terms will be loaded and encounters will be tracked to monitor financial performance.
- **Contract management.** Application components to support contract management include contract administration, decision support, and cost accounting. This process is typically where "nonrisk" contracts are managed.
- **Clinical and financial information management.** Various application components supporting information management include provider profiling, HEDIS reporting, data warehousing, and data access.
- **Network administration.** This process and its enabling application components are at the heart of what the network manager must accomplish—developing and administering multiple, large, and complex virtual provider delivery networks. Application components here include credentialing, provider demographics, and provider contracts.

Migration Issues

HCOs must establish an evolutionary migration path to reach the goal of network management. A good way to think about this is to examine the development levels through which HCOs progress as they respond to the growth of managed care in the marketplace. In the initial stages, HCOs begin to accept managed care contracts, typically discount and/or per diem arrangements.

The next step is usually the formation or a more formal provider contracting network encompassing hospitals, physicians, and outpatient providers and allowing for "single signature" contracts. Health systems will then begin to take risk in selected areas by developing "carve-outs," or centers of excellence in particular clinical areas like behavioral health, cardiovascular, orthopedics, and pediatrics. *The biggest leap will be when HCOs begin to accept broader capitation contracts, a move that will trigger significant process and technology changes required by network managers.* The final development stage will occur when an HCO enters into the health plan business directly by creating an insurance component to the integrated delivery network, such as a health maintenance organization (HMO) product for commercial, Medicaid, or Medicare.

Table 8.2 illustrates these development stages, along with the typical business triggers.

Transformation Issues

HCOs also face significant transformation issues in their evolution to the network manager role.

- **There must be balance established among the investments in clinical, acute, ambulatory, enterprise, and managed care systems.** Many healthcare orga-

TABLE 8.2. Development stages and typical business triggers.

Development stage	Business triggers
Contract administration	• Accepting discounted and per diem managed care contracts
Network management	• Developing formalized provider contracting network via physician hospital organization (PHO), MSO, etc., structure
	• Signing "simple signature" contracts
Focused intervention	• Accepting carve-out contacts
	• Developing center of excellence products
Capitation administration	• Accepting risk contracts with withholds and/or bonuses
	• Taking forms of capitation—global, physician, facility, primary care provider, etc.
	• Taking Medicaid or Medicare risk
Health plan product administration	• Functioning as a Medicare PSO
	• Operating a commercial, Medicare, individual/family, and/or Medicaid HMO

© First Consulting Group 1998

nizations overinvest in clinical and acute care systems while underinvesting in their managed care and ambulatory areas. The successful network manager must strike the right investment balance. An HCO must be able to balance the strategic risk of supporting managed care operations against the operational risk of supporting patient care systems. There is a trade-off here between continuing in the patient care role versus the long-term need to function as a network manager.

- **Managed care must be represented at the governance table of the HCO.** Most healthcare organizations have a vice president or director of managed care who is charged with the responsibility of marketing, network development, and contracting. This position typically does not represent managed care at the highest decision-making levels. It is crucial that managed care interests are represented in HCO executive management.
- **HCOs must own or control all critical medical management, financial, and capitation management processes, systems, and data.** These managed care processes and systems must be able to function at the network level as opposed to individual components for hospital, physician, and outpatient. Giving up control of these critical infrastructure elements can threaten the HCO and erode the core competencies necessary for network managers to function. This is imperative for the HCO accepting any type of risk contract—medical management responsibility should "flow with the risk."
- **Managed care systems must be deployed with a system-wide or network-wide view of the world.** Systems designed to support a network manager tend to cross departmental and functional lines. Historically, processes and systems for HCOs have operated along "departmental silos" such as patient accounting, lab, radiology, and admitting. Because of this, the development and implementation of network management systems must be in the hands of individuals who have the ability to take a network-wide view and can successfully resolve interdepartmental issues. This also implies that systems deployment must have the full support of executive management within the HCO in order to avoid "turf battles" that can potentially derail implementation.
- **Building the network management infrastructure is a complex, risky, time-consuming, and expensive endeavor.** Because of their complexity, the processes and systems must be developed in an incremental fashion. Integration, however, must be planned and maintained for each of the components as it is deployed. For example, if medical management capabilities are implemented first, the organization must consider how they will integrate with future claims and encounter administration needs. Timesharing, facilities management, and outsourcing options should be considered here as interim and/or long-term solutions for non-strategic functions. For instance, an organization may wish to outsource claims payment but not core medical management activities.
- **Data from multiple transaction systems must be combined to create integrated clinical and financial information.** This implies that data must be taken from existing clinical and financial systems such as patient accounting or med-

ical records and combined with new sources of managed care data such as claims and medical management systems. The data must then be "joined" and placed into common data warehouses to create uniform reports for provider profiling, HEDIS, etc.

Creating the Network Management Infrastructure

As an organization develops and implements the network manager model, it can learn lessons from other HCOs:

- Most HCOs currently lack the ability and capital to develop strategically significant managed care processes and systems to support this new role. Although payers do have these systems, they do not understand patient care processes and clinical data.
- Relying on payer partners for data does not work. Payers do not aggregate and report on data that supports provider medical manager activities. Their data are employer-oriented and lack data elements that are important to providers.
- Despite what is stated in sales presentations or seen in the latest brochures, *no vendor can provide a complete set of integrated managed care applications.* Systems from various vendors must be interfaced to provide a complete solution for the network manager needs.
- Small-scale sets of managed care applications can prove inadequate over time. These systems can perform well during a startup operation but trap the HCO in the long run because of their lack of functional depth and breadth, integration, and ability to handle increasing volumes of data.
- The new demands for technology support of new areas such as managed care and management service organizations (MSOs) are placing increased demands on an already strained IT delivery capability. Existing patient care and clinical systems tend to be inadequate and lack integration. Layering on new requirements for managed care and physician systems has placed HCOs in a perpetual catch-up mode.

Performance Metrics and Measurement Systems

Any new way of doing business requires new performance metrics and measurement systems that can track and report on performance. Healthcare purchasers have responded to inconsistent quality and pricing concerns with the delivery system by introducing new measures. The most widely recognized managed care measures are currently those developed by the National Committee for Quality Assurance (NCQA)–HEDIS. In the current version, HEDIS 3.0, the measures are broken down into multiple areas. Table 8.3 illustrates these areas along with some of the sample measures.

TABLE 8.3. HEDIS 3.0 measures.

Measurement area	Sample measures
Effectiveness of care	• Prenatal care in first trimester • Breast cancer screening • Flu shots for high-risk adults
Access to/availability of care	• Appointment access • Telephone access • Initiation of prenatal care
Member satisfaction	• Annual member health care survey
Health plan stability	• Member disenrollment • Physician turnover • Financial indicators
Use of services	• Inpatient utilization • Well-child visits in first 15 months of life • Cesarean section and rates of vaginal births after cesareans • Chemical dependency utilization
Cost of care	• High-occurrence/high-cost diagnosis related groups • Rate trends
Informed health choices	• New member education/orientation • Language translation
Healthcare delivery	• M.D. board certification • Family planning services • Quality assessment and improvement • Case management

HMO organizations such as the North Central Texas HEDIS Coalition are now compiling and reporting on HEDIS measures across multiple HMOs in the respective market. Some states—Texas, for example—are also mandating that HEDIS data be submitted on a statewide basis by HMOs.

Other emerging measurement systems include the Foundation for Accountability (FACCT) and the Joint Commission on Accreditation of Healthcare Organizations (JCAHO). FACCT, which currently represents more than 70 million members, was established as a public-private partnership by organizations like HCFA, the Department of Defense, the American Association of Retired Persons, American Express, and GTE. Organized to go beyond HEDIS and develop metrics that measure quality and outcomes of care, FACCT identifies, endorses, and promotes measures of quality and outcomes of care provided within health plans. FACCT's first measurement efforts focus on the following disease states:

- Depression
- Coronary artery disease
- Asthma
- Arthritis
- Breast cancer
- Coronary risk factor reduction

- Diabetes, hypertension
- Low back pain
- Pregnancy/maternity

JCAHO's Indicator Measurement System (IMSystem) is another comparative performance measurement database and system. The IMSystem is designed to measure organizational peformance, stimulate improved patient care, and generate reports on quality for patients, purchasers, and regulators. The system includes 42 indicators focusing on high-risk, high-volume, and high-cost areas of patient care, including:

- Obstetrics
- Cardiovascular care
- Oncology care
- Trauma care
- Medication use
- Infection control
- Anesthesia-related care.

The general network management principles presented here will lead to success, but we believe the rewards will be greatest for the HCOs that quickly embrace these concepts and successfully integrate them into their organizations and the patient care process. Those who ignore these network manager concepts will risk losing their core patient care business volumes to HCOs that move aggressively to develop a network manager capability. HCOs should march ahead boldly, unafraid to risk the possibility of setbacks and errors. To quote Theodore Roosevelt: "At a moment of decision, the best thing to do is the right thing; the next-best is the wrong thing; the worst thing to do is nothing."

References

Health Insurance Association of America. 1996. *Source Book of Health Insurance Data, 1995*. Washington, D.C.: Health Insurance Association of America.

Health Insurance Association of America. 1997. *Source Book of Health Insurance Data, 1996*. Washington, D.C.: Health Insurance Association of America.

Mullen, J.K. 1995. *Introduction to Managed Care: Fundamentals of Managed Care Coverage and Providers*. Atlanta, Ga.: LOMA.

Part 3

Enabling Technologies

9

Information Integration

TIM WEBB AND DALE WILL

Health care is undergoing many fundamental paradigm shifts. Most of these shifts in process are driving the demand for timely, reliable access to a preponderance of clinical information contained in different formats (paper and electronic), information systems, and locations. This has placed access to "one-stop shopping" for information at the forefront of most delivery network goals. The delivery of an integrated source of information has been as elusive as the pot of gold at the end of the rainbow. It has been attempted by several healthcare organizations but accomplished only rarely. As indicated by a recent benchmarking study of 40 integrated delivery networks (IDNs) (Figure 9.1), the level of clinical and operational information integration is, at best, just beginning. None of the participants indicated they had achieved the desired level of integration.

To help clear some of the fog that has enveloped information integration, this chapter will offer (a) a concise definition of what information integration is, (b) mechanisms for achieving integration, (c) a look at the challenges along the way, and (d) some insight into the process.

Information integration, rapidly becoming a catch-all "buzz word," will assuredly be expanded so that it too can have its own Three Letter Acronym (TLA). The computer world is whipping interest in information integration into a frenzy. Out of this will evolve some new and fantastic tools, along with many false starts and failed attempts. Although the goal of an integrated information environment is high on the priority list for many organizations, using a structured methodology to plan the integration is the challenge eluding most information services departments.

Defining Information Integration

Information integration has existed as a concept for many years, though it has gone by many different names. Simply put, information integration is the joining of business process and information systems. James Martin calls this process "information engineering." In the introduction to his book *Information Engineering*, he defines the process as: "an interlocking set of automated techniques in which

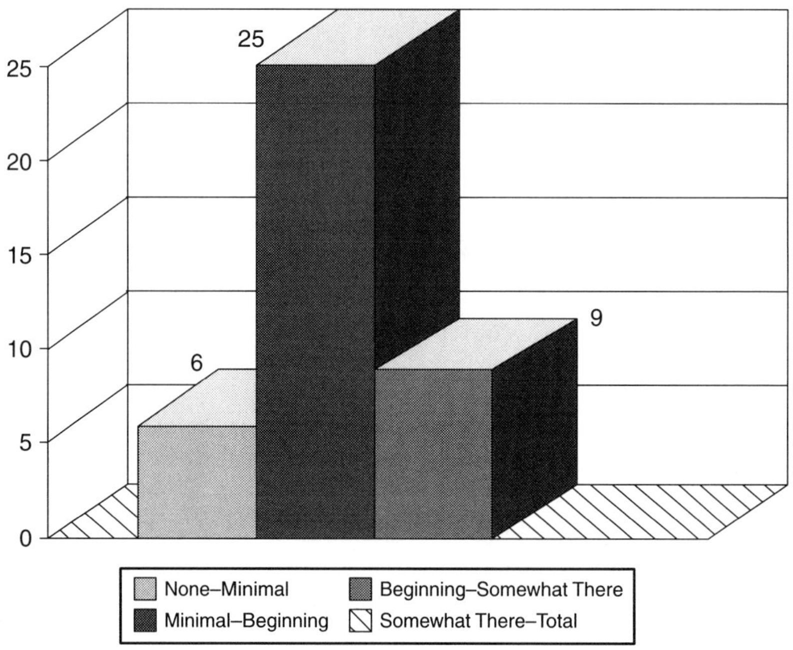

FIGURE 9.1. Level of Information Integration
© First Consulting Group 1997.

enterprise models, data models, and process models are built up in a comprehensive knowledge base and are used to create and maintain data processing systems" (1989, p. 1). To this end, we offer the following definition for health care:

Information integration is the process of bringing together disparate sources of clinical, financial, and other healthcare-related data in order to give the end user uniform access to all sources of information necessary to perform the job.

In health care, the requirements for predominant opportunities for integrated information are:

- unique identification of members within a population
- integrated patient registry
- unified problem lists
- clinical decision support
- access to eligibility information
- seamless communication with other providers
- analysis of costs and outcomes across various settings.

This definition has several implications. First, given the state of healthcare information technology, no single vendor can offer a packaged solution to meet all of these requirements for any one end user, let alone an entire customer base.

Second, though the definition gives tangible boundaries, it also implies a significant amount of work will be required to implement integrated information solutions. This is a tall order for most information services departments. Also, other clinical and nonclinical departments will need to evaluate their processes in order to reap the benefits of integrated information. This will require changes in process and the collection of clinical information.

Along with a definition for information integration, information services must have uniform definitions for many other terms. The following is a series of definitions for some of the "hot" topics (this is not an exhaustive list):

- **Clinical data repository**—an operational data store that contains patient-centered information, is updated real-time or near real-time, and is organized for quick retrieval.
- **Data warehouse**—a data store used for analysis and reporting of aggregated views of the clinical and financial performance of the enterprise.
- **Data mining**—a method of searching data for hidden patterns or relationships using a variety of tools and algorithms (Devlin 1997).
- **Data modeling**—the process of formally documenting the data needs of users and the database structures required to satisfy those needs (Devlin 1997).
- **Interface engine**—a product that allows disparate types of systems to directly share data with each other at the application layer.
- **Standards organizations**—groups of individuals, companies, and providers that develop specifications for passing information between disparate systems. These groups are usually accredited by organizations like the American National Standards Institute (ANSI) or International Standards Organization (ISO). Other examples are Health Level 7 (HL7), X12n and Arden Syntax, and Common Object Request Brokering Architecture (CORBA).

The Current Horizon: Clinical Data Repositories and Data Warehouses

When organizations ask how information integration is achieved, two types of information storage mechanisms come to mind: the clinical data repository (CDR) and the data warehouse. In today's world, both of these information storage mechanisms are usually based on a relational database design and are deployed on either Sybase or Oracle relational database management system (RDBMS). Both mechanisms, however, serve vastly different purposes relative to the enterprise's information needs.

Clinical Data Repositories

As previously stated, CDRs are operational data stores (databases) that contain patient-centered information designed for quick retrieval of that information. In addition, they are usually recipients of information from feeder or ancillary systems rather than generators of information. CDRs can be the ultimate "garbage in–garbage out" systems since they are dependent on the data quality from ancillary systems. This provides a strong argument for evaluating the data quality and quantity relative to the ancillary systems.

As Figure 9.2 illustrates, end users interact with various transaction systems, sometimes referred to as the ancillary or feeder systems. This interaction includes entering and retrieving data from the various sources. When data are entered into one of these transaction systems—for example, admission information from the admission/discharge/transfer (ADT) registration system—an electronic package of data is generated upon completion of a data entry session. This package of data is sent via a network to the integration tools, e.g., interface engine. The integration tools then perform some consistency and quality checks as well as reformatting the data package into the site's information transmission standard, e.g., HL7. The package is then forwarded to the appropriate receiving systems. As shown in Figure 9.2, the clinical data repository is one of the prime recipients of this data package. In a similar fashion, requests for information are usually generated at the caregiver workstation and transmitted to the integration tools via a network. The integration tools route the query to the appropriate database,

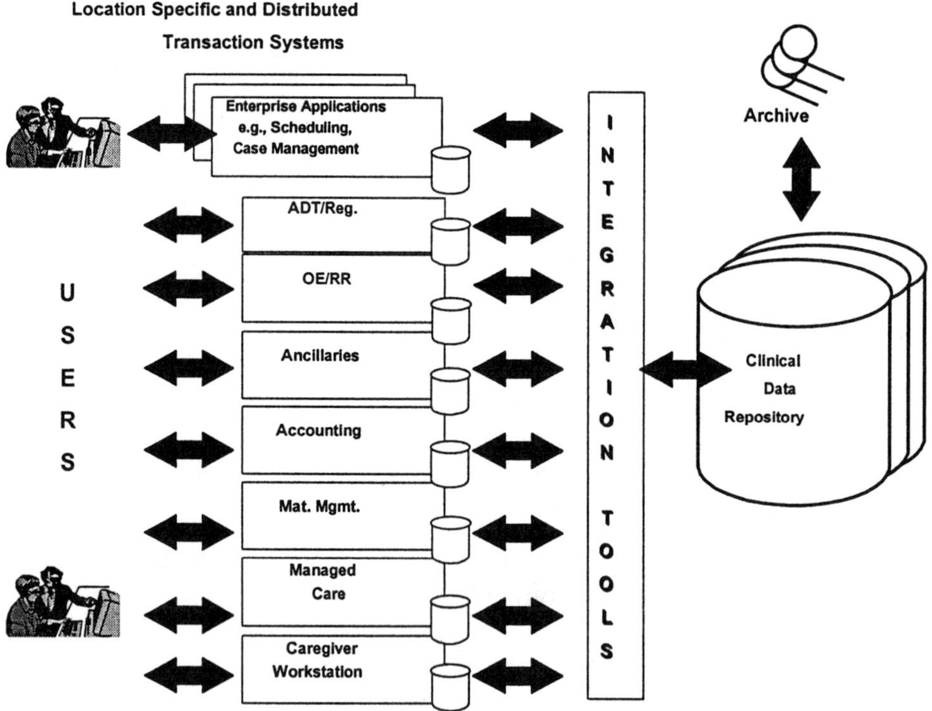

FIGURE 9.2. Deployed Data Repository
© First Consulting Group 1997.

e.g., clinical data repository, where the request is fulfilled and information is returned to the workstation.

There are many uses for a well-deployed clinical data repository. For example, a CDR can provide longitudinal views of patient information. Data repositories are usually organized primarily around patients and secondly around visits or encounters, a method of organization that easily accommodates views that span multiple visits. This type of view allows clinicians to trend and chart results independent of the visits and test panel organization. For example, a clinician could study the trend of a patient's blood sodium levels over the past six months independent of what types of panels or batteries originated the result.

CDRs also provide access to information where it is needed. Since they receive information from a multitude of feeder systems, well-deployed CDRs can create a "one-stop shopping" environment. This is done by allowing the clinical staff to access a variety of patient-focused information through a consistent and (it is hoped) easy-to-use graphical user interface (GUI). The GUI access can be deployed through hand-held devices, bedside computing devices, computers in physician offices, or computing devices deployed at nursing stations. In any case, this wide variety of information access moves far closer to deployment of information at the point of care.

Finally, CDRs offer a cross-continuum view of information, since they allow information to be gathered and viewed from sources other than an acute setting. This type of ambulatory-focused information combines with the acute information to give clinicians a new level of insight into the wellness of their patients. The CDR is leading the way in providing this cross-continuum view.

Data Warehouses

Like CDRs, data warehouses provide a different "look" at clinical and financial information. Data quality issues are still pertinent when deploying a data warehouse. Figure 9.3 shows how the components interact in a deployed data warehouse.

The data warehouse operates very similarly to the clinical data warehouse (see explanation preceding Figure 9.2 for detail). The fundamental difference is that the data warehouse is updated in a batch mode, i.e., data packages are queued and inserted en masse as opposed to real-time. This may require the integration tools to route the data packets to a site-specific queuing mechanism. This queuing mechanism holds the data packages until the jobs for batch loading the warehouse are executed.

A healthcare-oriented data warehouse has many practical uses. For instance, it is capable of cross-patient population searches. Though data warehouses gather information similar to that of a CDR (with perhaps a bit more financial information), they organize this information in a vastly different fashion. One way to organize the information takes away the patient-centered view and provides a cross-population view. This approach allows for queries such as "Give me the number of magnetic resonance imagings performed from 1/1/96 to 5/1/96 for pa-

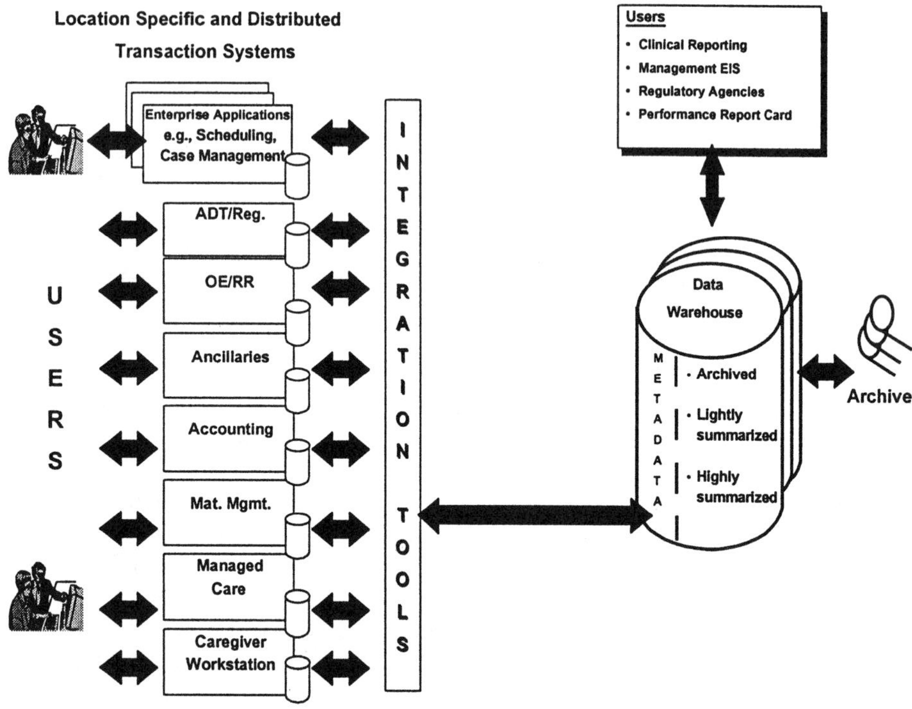

FIGURE 9.3. A Deployed Data Warehouse
© First Consulting Group 1997.

tients living in ZIP codes 15907, 15908, and 15905." Queries like these span patient populations and usually require a different database structure (or, at minimum, a different indexing structure).

At the forefront of most enterprises is the analysis of outcomes and the ensuing development of best practices or protocols. A properly organized data warehouse can provide this kind of information by allowing queries such as "Give me the discharge disposition of my patients with a diagnosis of pneumonia, not otherwise specified, that received penicillin within 24 hours of admitting." This class of query can reveal a great deal of information and provide a springboard for further drill-down and analysis.

The data warehouse can also provide answers to analyses of actual cost versus reimbursed or capitated costs. This can be done with queries as simple as "Give me the number of complete blood counts performed over the past six months." In its simplest form, the query could provide a raw number that could be plugged into a very simple calculation using the current charge master. In essence, a well-organized and populated data warehouse can easily provide a wealth of information about an enterprise's financial performance.

In addition, data warehouses make the process of data mining easier. As previously defined, data mining looks for less-than-obvious relationships among the collected data. For example, an extraordinarily high percentage of patients who are diagnosed with appendicitis and placed in nursing unit 4W might return within two weeks of discharge with a severe headache. Retailing provides another classic example of "hidden relationships": it is often believed that if diapers are placed by the beer cooler, many more men than usual will buy diapers when they are purchasing beer (or the other way around). In any case, a data warehouse provides a sound information foundation for data mining.

When designed and implemented correctly, both clinical data repositories and data warehouses can provide significant benefits. Executives must remember, however, that these two storage mechanisms are still relatively new to the healthcare arena. Despite the last decade's technological triumphs, there are still very few experts in clinical data repositories and virtually none in healthcare-oriented data warehousing. For this reason, the executives should have a very critical eye on the employee or consultant who claims expert-level knowledge in these areas.

Tomorrow's Sunrise: Promising Technologies

Implementing clinical data repositories and data warehouses typically requires new processes and technologies for collecting and retrieving clinical data. The advent of new technologies has enhanced the value of data warehouse technology, based on the synergy it provides when combined with new processes. Two of the more visible technologies are smart cards and hand-held computers.

Smart Cards

Smart cards are the size of credit cards and contain a small memory chip that stores basic medical information. As technology improves, the chip might be able to store a patient's entire medical history. Although smart cards are rarely seen in the United States, Europe uses them widely to support nationalized healthcare systems. About 55 million people in Germany are already using smart cards in this way, and similar systems are about to emerge in France and possibly the United Kingdom (Emig 1997). Smart cards can provide many benefits and opportunities, but there are a few caveats. Potential problems with smart cards include keeping the data secure and consolidating and storing all the data on the card somewhere else in case of loss or damage to the card.

Hand-Held Computers

Hand-held computers will help deliver information at the exact point of care. An article in the *Computerworld Health Care Journal* illustrated the potential benefits of this burgeoning technology. In the article, nurses at the Visiting Nurse Service of New York briefly tuned in to how their professional lives would change if they could scrap overstuffed patient record folders in favor of hand-held computers equipped with wireless modems. "All of the patient chart and demographic information I needed was accessible to me," said Deborah Freeman, an registered nurse with the not-for-profit home health giant. "It was wonderful" (Watson 1996, p. 18). The biggest issue with this technology is how to adapt existing graphical user interfaces written for a 15-inch screen to a small hand-held screen.

Critical Success Factors

One of the key success factors is understanding that the development of an integrated information environment usually is not just a technical project. Rather, it is an organizational vision and objective. Providing an integrated information environment is not easy, simply because it transcends barriers—real and imagined—across the enterprise. Creating this type of environment will stretch the skill sets of even the most astute and well-developed information services department, but the demand and need are real and must be accomplished. Since access to integrated information can focus the whole enterprise, the result of these efforts can be amazing.

To achieve information integration, the executive management must make sure their strategy includes:

- **Proper organizational structure and support.** The first step toward success is to ensure executive management support and a solid organization structure. This is necessary in order to support the many enterprise-wide initiatives needed to provide an integrated information environment. Figure 9.4 illustrates one approach to a possible organization structure.

  Proper organization is crucial. According to a March 1996 Gartner Group Report, "less than 50 percent of the potential return [of IT investments] flow through the enterprise—inappropriate management practices and work organization for the deployed IT absorbs the balance."
- **Automated tools and methodologies.** Developing the complex business process, entity relationship, and data models requires sophisticated tools. These tools must be integrated and capable of being translated for use by the application developers.
- **End user focus with a healthy dose of input from the physician community.** In most cases, information integration projects are rooted in the need to provide appropriate information to appropriate users at an appropriate time. Usually one of the larger, harder-to-please end-user communities is the physicians. It is vital for projects involving integration of data sources to gain the confidence and support of the physicians. This can be done in many ways. For instance, they might be invited to the governance/advisory boards, included as subject matter experts, or involved in vendor selection processes.

  Physicians tend to have the most intensive and varied needs for information. If a project does not satisfy their needs, it is usually deemed a failure. Conversely, if the project does meet the needs of the physician community, it is called a resounding success.

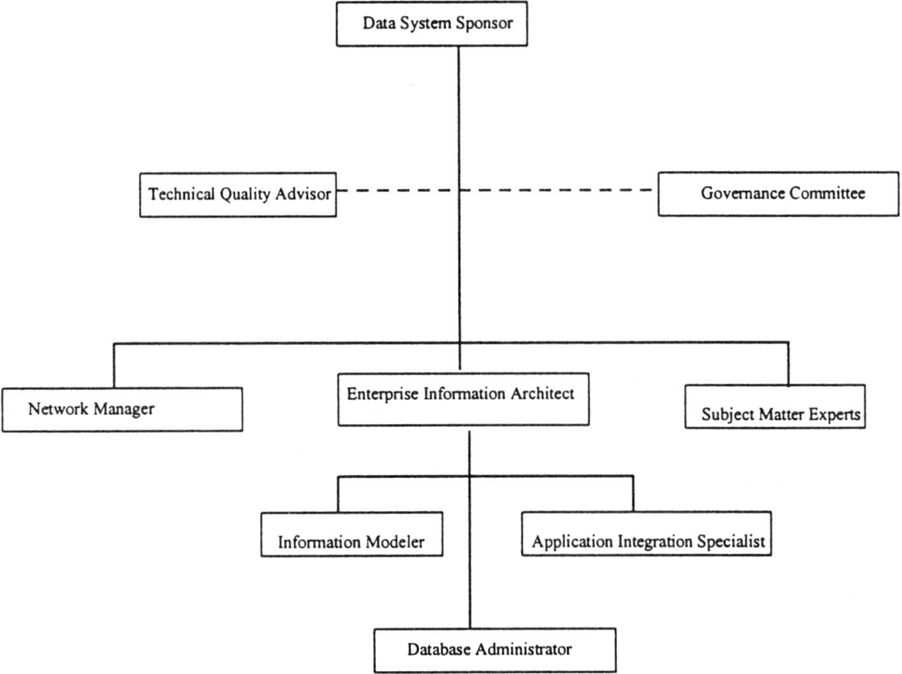

FIGURE 9.4. Organization Structure
© First Consulting Group 1997.

- **Change readiness.** Successful information integration strategies are dependent on reengineering from department processes to cross-continuum processes. These types of changes are radical and often politically sensitive. The reason for this is simple: this type of project is usually the first to span the enterprise and all of the real and "virtual" walls. Executive management must agree to support the interests of the enterprise over individual business unit priorities when it comes to changed processes. Lack of overriding leadership to resolve political skirmishes is the main reason information integration projects fail.
- **Standards for passing information and data element definitions.** Data standards are a critical element of information integration. An early step for any enterprise attempting to develop and deploy an information integration strategy is the development of standards across the enterprise. Standards will help lower the cost of interfaces between systems and provide a sound basis for uniform access to a single source of information.

  These standards come at several levels, but two key areas are information transmission and data definitions. In the areas of information transmission, HL7 (clinical), X12n (financial), National Council for Prescription Drug Programs (NCPDP) (drugs), and Digital Imaging and Communications in Medicine (DICOM) (images) are the leaders in their areas of specialty. Regarding data definitions, also called controlled vocabularies or lexicons, groups such as Systematized Nomenclature of Medicine (SNOMED) and Logical Observation Identifiers, Names and Codes (LOINC) are leaders.

The area of standards and controlled vocabularies present the biggest challenge in health care. The lack of standards has greatly impaired most efforts regarding information integration. Notwithstanding the level of effort required to adopt standards, doing so will save the enterprise much more effort in the long run.

- **Proper budgeting.** An information integration strategy requires investment, in terms of both money and time. Budgetary estimates range from several hundred thousand to several millions, and time estimates are from six months to five years. These projects can be substantial over several years, so the best approach is an incremental one. Do not try to tackle the enterprise top to bottom initially. Continued investments over a sustained period will reap greater long-term benefits.
- **In-depth understanding of the enterprise's business processes and shortcomings.** This is absolutely key to the success of any project or strategy involving information integration. Information integration can provide a rallying point to drive the evaluation and possible modification of an enterprise's business process (e.g., admissions, billing). The executive management of the enterprise must seize this opportunity. It is important to remember that placing new technology on ineffective or inappropriate business processes will negatively impact the value of an information integration approach.
- **Expectation management.** It is a true balancing act to maintain a high level of end-user involvement in order to get end-user buy-in, but maintain a reasonable level of expectation about what will be delivered. Remember, successful projects crawl before they walk and walk before they run. For example, if a clinical data repository project is in progress or envisioned, the pilot project functionality must be limited. It is fine to announce that the data repository will give access to various images, patient-centered ADT, financial and pharmacy information, order management, result reporting, and clinical decision support, but this list sets the user's expectations extraordinarily high. The probability of the information services department being able to deliver this in less than two years is near zero. It would be better if the management team announced that an integrated source of information initially containing ADT and results reporting using a well-designed, flexible GUI will be available in nine months; a timeline spelling out additional functionality and release dates could also be distributed. Since the user's expectations would be reasonable, this project would have a much higher probability of success. Unmanaged user expectation is the death knell of a project.
- **Security, confidentiality, and privacy strategy in place.** Although the exact requirements are in flux, it is safe to say that security, confidentiality, and privacy policies must be at the forefront of an information integration strategy. Two suggested World Wide Web information sites to be monitored for up-to-

the-minute information are http://aspe.os.dhhs.gov/admnsimp/ and http://aspe.os.dhhs.gov/ncvhs/.

- **Long-ranging view and vision of health care as a whole and of the specific enterprise.** One area that is often given insufficient attention is the need for a strategic vision for the enterprise. At minimum, this strategic vision includes the corporate vision, a mission statement, a technology architecture, and an information architecture. These combine to form the cornerstone by which successes in information integration strategies can be measured. In addition to being a cornerstone by which to measure success, the strategic vision will be used in driving vendor choices and deployment strategies, resolving conflicts, and generally helping the enterprise maintain its focus.

Process for Implementation

Implementing information integration is a simple process based on surprisingly old principles. Information processing is thousands of years old; only the technology is new. The concepts of Greek philosophers Plato and Aristotle are pertinent today as we attempt to classify the data and relationships required to deliver quality health care. Classification theory and object-oriented analysis are key to developing integrated systems.

The process of information integration planning starts during the strategic information management planning process. The strategic planning process should focus on the key business processes and high-level data architecture. As the organization agrees on the priorities of the business, the need for integration is focused on specific business processes and information systems. In some cases, the result of this strategic planning is not the need for new applications, but the need to integrate existing applications.

The next step is to focus on a process, like access to care. As part of redesigning access to care, information integration is tackled as a series of discrete but integrated tasks. These tasks are focused on identifying the detailed workflow, current and future, using automated tools. Simultaneously, a data dictionary and data model should be built to correspond to the process being redesigned.

The next phase is to develop detailed designs that will provide the integration necessary to support the new business processes. The design process is greatly condensed if automated tools have been used during the initial phases. The detail design may specify implementation of interface engines, data warehouses, and possibly new enterprise-wide applications to replace legacy applications focused on a single department.

The final phase is to implement the solutions. With automated tools, there is little room for surprises and issues. In addition, the implementation effort can be condensed through the use of integrated design and development tools. If the scope of work addressed is discrete enough, an effort such as this can easily be achieved in 12 to 18 months. An example is the Veterans Health Administration, where this basic process is being followed. The project will result in the largest enrollment and registration system in the United States. Based on a highly complex architecture integrating legacy applications with a myriad of data warehouses, the system will be capable of enrolling 28 million veterans.

Recommendations for the CEO

As with any project in any arena, there are certain steps a CEO can take to move the project along in a much easier fashion. At minimum, any CEO developing an information integration strategy should:

- Assess the environment to make sure executive management is in this for the long haul.
- Make sure the process is integrated with the business's strategic plan.
- Tackle a discrete project with information integration; do not take on the enterprise.
- Make sure money is available with a contingency fund—more than likely, costs will exceed initial estimates of time and money.
- Monitor progress closely to make sure timelines and budgets are within reason and are being met.
- Verify that the information systems department understands the complexities of information integration, and expect to bring in outside expertise to facilitate the process.
- Insist on industry-accepted methodologies and approaches for software and information engineering.
- Insist on using automated tools for business process and data modeling.
- Insist on adopting standards.
- Expect some bumps to occur and be ready to deal with a high level of frustration—this is a new technology and approach for the healthcare information system.
- Provide an ample training budget for technical staff and end users.
- Read, read, read, and make sure the management team is conversant about current technology.

We're on the brink of one of the biggest changes we'll see. Today in the Brigham, and about to go into the General, is a home-grown system whereby all medication orders are written on the computer. Every day, out of 13,000, 380 are changed because the computer says the patient is allergic to that drug, the prescribed dose is too large, that drug interacts with another drug, the lab test you ordered is unnecessary. The issue we have is managing the vast amount of knowledge. We have 2,500 drugs available, 1,500 laboratory tests, hundreds of diagnoses—the mind is not capable of containing that information, but it's nothing for the computer. (Dr. H. Richard Nesson, former President of Partners Healthcare, quoted in *The Boston Globe Magazine,* [Koch, 1997, p. 14])

The deployment of an information integration system is a long and arduous process that transcends all real and virtual walls of the enterprise. Providing an environment of integrated information demands that business processes be evaluated and altered if necessary, political challenges be addressed head-on and resolved, and standards be chosen and adopted across the enterprise. The task at hand is certainly not easy, but the results of deploying a well-planned information integration strategy will improve the delivery of care across the enterprise and, in the long run, ensure its longevity.

References

First Consulting Group. 1997. "Creating the 21st Century Integrated Delivery Network, Current Status and Emerging Models," *Emerging Practices*, White Paper, Long Beach, Calif.: FCG.

Devlin, B. 1997. *Data Warehouse from Architecture to Implementation*. Reading, Mass.: Addison-Wesley.

Koch, J. "Interview with H. Richard Nesson." 1997. *Boston Globe Magazine*, September, p. 14.

Martin, J. 1989. *Information Engineering*, Book I: Introduction. New York: Prentice Hall.

Emig, J. "Smart Card Use to Reach 2.3 Billion by Year 2001." 1997. *Newsbytes News Network*, September 3. Available on http://www.newbytes.com/news/97

Watson, S. "Sounding Out Wireless." 1996. *Computerworld Health Care Journal*, October 1, p. 18.

10

Application Development

TOM HURLEY AND MICHAEL FEYEN

Today's information technology (IT) managers must contend with many difficult issues when deciding on the best approach to developing mission-critical, enterprise-wide software applications. It is more important than ever for high-performance IT organizations to develop cost-effective, quality solutions while maintaining the flexibility to compete in the dynamic, always changing world of applications development. The pressure IT managers face is considerable, since the role the IT organization plays within a company can determine the methods by which applications are developed.

If the IT function is viewed as an enabler of strategic development, then it may be advantageous to keep a nucleus of quality staff on board and look to outsource some or all major development efforts. If the IT staff is considered a core functionality within a business and is counted on to develop and maintain the product set, it becomes critical to define a good internal development process and infrastructure.

In this chapter, we will discuss some of the benefits of external product development and some key elements to pinpoint when outsourcing development to a third-party vendor. We will also describe some good internal development practices to follow when building products and demonstrate how these practices can benefit an organization.

External Development: Outsourcing

As companies continue to experience competitive pressures to cut product and development costs without compromising standards of quality, more and more organizations are outsourcing their application development projects. We believe that outsourcing all or selected aspects of applications development and maintenance can actually accelerate the value realized from IT investments. This is reinforced by the fact that applications development and maintenance outsourcing are, respectively, the first and second most frequently outsourced IT activities.

Cost and resource constraints are the key factors behind the decision to outsource applications development and maintenance. The major factors include:

- Operating expenses can be reduced or controlled.
- Resources can be redirected for other strategic initiatives.
- The required resources are not available within the organization.
- Outsourcing maintenance work allows more time for new development.
- Migrating from legacy systems to new platforms requires new skill-sets.

The potential benefits of outsourcing development projects are numerous. For instance, outsourcing ensures that expert consultants are available to meet the changing needs of the project and predict skill-set requirements. External development can provide a cost-effective resource utilization alternative; it can also bring new and fresh ideas to the group. *If it is planned well and for the right reasons, outsourcing can improve the competitiveness and flexibility of any IT organization.*

Outsourcing Agents

The process of determining when to outsource and which vendor to enlist can be daunting. For guidance, a business might hire outsourcing agents—technology companies and consultants who help organizations decide when to outsource and to whom. We believe outsourcing agents are ideal for IT organizations burdened by insufficient time, people, or skills to evaluate the potential benefits and risks of outsourcing. Some of the services that agents provide are:

- **Requests for proposals (RFPs)/contract writing.** This includes developing RFPs and reviewing vendor responses.
- **Cost/benefit analysis.** This entails providing an estimate of the potential revenue enhancement or cost reduction associated with a project.
- **Contract management.** Managing the vendor's activities after the contract has been signed is a significant effort that includes overseeing the vendor's work and renegotiating terms and/or ending contracts.
- **Technology assessments.** Agents can evaluate the risks of staying with a current product set and determine the cost and risk of going to new technologies.
- **Vendor selection.** This includes an evaluation of vendors to narrow the available choices to those that would best serve the project's needs.

Managing External Development

Once the vendor has been selected and the contract signed, managing the project becomes the primary task. Managing external development projects from start to finish can be difficult, but IT management can help ensure success by focusing on a few specific areas.

First, IT managers should develop a procedure to handle contract changes. Altering an original contract is one of the most delicate procedures to manage; on fixed-price contracts, each change can increase the risk and cost to the vendor. Change, however, is also a fact of life and a crucial component of a project's success. For this reason, IT managers need to keep the vendor open to new possibilities by effectively managing the change control process.

This process should begin while both parties are planning the contract, which can be the change agent that helps define the parameters of product development. A contract should be flexible enough to please the vendor, but it should still provide enough checkpoints and specifics to protect the business from unfinished or unsatisfactory work. Managers must remember that vendors, who are focused on making a profit, may not be interested in altering their plan of action to increase the product's value to the end user. Well-structured contracts can define the objectives in a way that will keep vendors happy while motivating them to produce a product that will surpass expectations. If both sides can follow the spirit of the contract, then change can be easier to control and implement, objectives will be met, and conflict will be lessened.

Before those objectives can be met, however, they must be clearly articulated. One sure way to invite trouble when outsourcing development projects is to miscommunicate goals. If one party fails to clarify its needs before the project is launched, they might begin with different objectives in mind, a problem that will leave the door open for conflict, wasted time and resources, and mutual disappointment. To ensure that their goals and the vendors' goals match, managers should get buy-in from the vendors as early as possible.

Because success often hinges on understanding what motivates the vendor, developing a good relationship, and keeping that relationship healthy, maintaining clear communication is crucial at all stages of the project. We suggest that IT managers have regular face-to-face project checkpoints with the vendor to make sure the contract is being interpreted correctly. A set of project deliverables at each phase of the project will help confirm that the project is moving along as it should and that the vendor is fulfilling the requirements. If the business desires another performance measure, an acceptance test plan is an excellent mechanism for determining that product functionality meets expectations.

As a final precaution, managers should transfer skills and knowledge to internal IT staff to lessen dependence on the vendor. The project will be more successful when the end users know how to use and support the product. *IT (and all end users) must assume ownership and be ready to run with the product when it is completed and ready for use.*

Common Development Pitfalls

Unfortunately, even the most skillful negotiation and communication cannot guarantee that the project will run smoothly. Whether a business is dealing with inhouse applications or external vendors, it may contend with problem areas that must be navigated with care if the project is to survive. Because unaddressed problems can result in project delays, cost overruns, or project failure, managers need to examine ways to prevent and solve them.

Underestimating Work Effort

Too often, development managers encounter projects that underestimate the time and resources required to build a product. Some things clearly are unavoidable: a tool vendor may go under, or key staff members may leave in mid-project. To keep the project on schedule, managers must account for these risks in the project plan and identify contingency plans early in the project. It is important (whenever possible) not to commit to schedules and deliverables until requirements and a high-level design are in place and approved by both parties. Spending the time and money to determine project scope prior to estimating complete project requirements for people, dollars, and end dates greatly lessens the risk of underestimating the project.

Tool Failure

Another problem is tool failure, or the inability of development tools to create the required system. To prevent this from happening, tools need to be tested before they are selected. With a requirements specification and high-level design in place, a business will be better equipped to select the proper tool set and methodology to accomplish its project goals. If problems with development tools cannot be overcome, a business should carefully select another tool to build the application.

Architecture Failure

Architecting the wrong solution for a problem can cause more serious problems. For instance, implementing a two-tiered client-server solution instead of a three-tiered solution can cause performance problems for high-volume online transaction processing (OLTP) network intensive applications. As in the tool failure problem, businesses need to identify the problem, create and test a new architecture, and head in a new direction.

Lack of Defined Development Process

A documented development process must be in place to effectively develop software. The rest of this chapter describes some industry-accepted practices, activities, and methods that can be adopted by any organization in pursuit of its quality-driven mission.

Internal Development

We believe the key to any successful development project is having the proper development process and infrastructure in place. A mission statement for many development organizations includes a vow to "produce products of the highest possible quality in a cost-effective, timely manner." *The only way in which quality, budget, and scheduling goals can be routinely met is through a disciplined approach to software development and maintenance.* This approach includes the creation of a development infrastructure to support the activities of the organization, as well as a defined, documented, repeatable, verifiable, and controlled process for developing software products.

Benefits of Development Standards

Before a business attempts to develop and implement new software, a set of standards should be created. Implementing software development standards can reduce costs and improve quality, set guidelines for training employees (giving them the tools to make decisions under generally defined criteria), and establish quality as a practice ingrained in the day-to-day activities of all development personnel. In addition, creating a well documented development process puts a business ahead when positioning itself for ISO 9000 certification. Implementing ISO 9000 standards helps increase the customers' confidence in the quality systems of their suppliers, stimulates continuous quality improvements, and provides the necessary tools to deliver consistent, controlled, and defect-free products.

The benefits derived from implementing development standards and processes (and becoming ISO 9000–certified) are numerous. Implementation can:

- allow companies to improve their processes, resulting in higher-quality products and services
- require companies to document what they do, not necessarily change what they do, and adhere to the documented quality procedures
- establish a "say what you do, do what you say, and prove that you did it" program
- result in significant improvement in overall operations effectiveness
- assure the customers that quality products are being developed.

Once a particular process is documented and accepted as the way in which a development organization will conduct business, half the battle is won. What remains is the task of managing projects in a way that enforces the developed processes. It is easy to "talk the talk." With good project management, proper review cycles, and efficient development tools, the development organization can "walk the walk," enforcing the processes put in place.

Developing Software

As in other engineering disciplines, a standardized approach can be applied to the development of software:

- Use of proven methods during each step in the development life cycle
- Use of reviews at various milestones to ensure quality

- Creation of specific documentation at each step
- Use of tools and methods to expedite development
- Traceability of all functionality in the finished product back to the original concept
- Creation of a change control process to control product scope
- Use of strong project management to help ensure adherence to standards and schedules.

The procedures, tools, standards, and processes adopted by an organization should include standardized development documents, a formal review methodology, coding standards and guidelines, rigorous product testing, source code control procedures, a design change control process, user documentation guidelines, a defect tracking system, and well-documented maintenance practices and procedures. These procedures and tools, when combined with effective project management and adherence to standards, provide the proper level of consistency, repeatability, control, and certification to product development efforts.

Standardized Development Documents

The use of standard documents for the software development process promotes common terminology and greatly eases the task of reviewing or researching by nonproject members or staff from other departments. Defining templates for requirements, high-level design documents, detailed-level design documents, unit, integration, validation, and system test plans helps promote consistency and repeatability across projects. It also helps enforce a standard process for the phases of development in which the documents are produced.

Documented procedures must be established and maintained to control and verify the design of the product and ensure that specified requirements are met. One of the keys to good design and test plan documentation is documenting all items in a way that can easily be cross-referenced and verified against product requirements. This means the items can be compared with the original product requirements and fully tested to ensure that those requirements are being met.

Formal Review Methodology

The most effective way to improve the quality of any product is removing defects as early in the development life cycle as possible. Numerous studies have shown that between 50 and 65 percent of all defects are introduced in the design phase of the development process. Other studies have indicated a dramatic increase in the cost of defect removal in later stages of the product life cycle. Formal technical reviews, conducted in an iterative fashion at each step in the development cycle, have proven to be the most effective weapon in exposing and correcting defects.

In addition to exposing defects, the review process also serves as the approval process. For example, once a document has exited its review cycle, it becomes an approved document. Once approved, a document becomes a baseline for further development work. Subsequent development should not occur until the previous process step is completed and the associated document is reviewed and approved.

Regular project reviews are also important review vehicles. Project reviews help assess project progress, current risks, and adherence to standards; in addition, they evaluate the overall quality of the project.

Coding Standards and Guidelines

Consistency and repeatability can also be promoted by establishing coding standards and guidelines. These standards are not meant to impose restrictions or limitations; rather, they are designed to improve the readability and efficiency of the source code, making it easier to understand and maintain. Coding standards can be enforced through informal peer reviews or formal code reviews, depending on the stage of development.

Product Testing

Product testing, both formal and informal, requires careful planning and preparation. Using standardized testing methods and documentation, project members should design a test plan that will produce quantifiable, verifiable results. Each test in the plan should aim to define the inputs, test steps, outputs, expected results, variations from expected results, and whether the test passed or failed. Once the plan is designed, actual testing should be conducted by a group other than the team that designed the system and wrote the code. The product will receive invaluable exposure from another group of software professionals experienced with the product, client base, and industry-accepted test procedures.

We believe rigorous product testing is the cornerstone of building quality products. The implementation of formal test plans will contribute to the overall software reliability, maintainability, and traceability; it will also improve the consistency of test documentation.

Source Code Control Procedures

Configuration management and source control tools are two other essential components of successful software development. Configuration management provides a mechanism for identifying, controlling, and tracking the versions of each software module. As modules mature through the development phases, they must be placed under source control to limit the possibility of overwriting changes.

Source control also provides a means for verifying and controlling changes to modules by keeping a revision history of all updates to the module. Placing design documentation and test plans under revision control is a way to maintain a history of all changes to design documents after the original sign-off on the documents.

Design Change Control Process

Change is a fact of life in the software development life cycle, and effective control over changes during all phases of development is a key concern of software developers. Without a clear estimation of the impact each proposed design change will have on work effort, schedule, and cost, managing software projects becomes almost impossible. If there is no way to identify, approve, and document all changes, the scope of the project increases, and the original documentation no longer reflects the finished product. This makes long-term maintenance difficult.

To effectively manage the constant change that occurs, we recommend an iterative approach to development. Each project phase must have a mechanism for identifying, documenting, and approving changes; if no mechanism exists, the project members might find themselves dealing with costly errors. For example, changing a design concept during implementation could easily result in changes to documents that already have been completed, which will require time-consuming backtracking.

Defect Tracking System

Defect tracking systems are vital to the success of any software development project. Exposed defects must be tracked and managed properly so that problems can be resolved as quickly and efficiently as possible.

A successful defect tracking and control system should:

- guarantee that exposed defects are corrected
- provide project members with automatic notification of problem status and assignment
- allow problems to be traced back to phases of development, which aids in quality control by pointing out problems in specific areas of development
- generate reports to track problem trends and assignments
- provide metrics that help predict current and future product quality.

Maintenance Practices and Procedures

As with other phases of the software development life cycle, standards and guidelines can be applied to the maintenance phase. All changes to the software made during the maintenance phase should be carried out in the same manner that the original product was developed. The changes should also be approved and documented according to the document control and configuration management procedures in place.

Implementation documents should be created for each problem. These documents should indicate the problem, responsible developer, subsystem affected, problem analysis, reference to an initial problem report, implementation description, modules modified, functions modified, and any additions to existing test plans that must be made because of the changes.

Project Management

Another key to successful software development is enlisting strong project managers to oversee the development efforts. A good project manager should:

- create a work breakdown structure, or list of the major tasks that must occur in order to build the product
- produce a project plan, consisting of a description of the project purpose, the resources needed (people, computers, etc.), tasks, deliverables, project risks, and a high-level schedule with dates for deliverables and end dates for project phases
- monitor the progress of the project and produce weekly status reports
- work with other project members and teams to coordinate and prioritize development efforts.

Because the project manager must get all members of the team to work together, he or she should allow (or even encourage) individuals to help other team members if there is an area of the project that is suffering. With the project manager's guidance, team members should learn to place overall team goals ahead of their individual goals. In doing so, team members will begin to help others, volunteer for additional work, and gain an understanding that their success as a team depends on the success of the whole project.

Project managers can also help ensure that established processes and controls are being followed. By properly managing each phase of development, managers can establish criteria (or gates) that must be met before product development can progress to the next phase. If these criteria are measurable and verifiable, the milestones and deliverables will give a valid indication of progress.

Certain tools are available to help project managers track progress, control product changes, and manage the activities of team members. A good project scheduling tool (such as Microsoft Project Manager) and a defect control system (such as Intersolv's PVCS Tracker) would be sound investments.

Development Support Groups

In order to fully support an organization's quality-driven mission, we believe a development infrastructure must be established to support the objectives of creating and adhering to the defined processes. This infrastructure should include the creation of the following groups or defined roles to support the development process:

- **Quality assurance group.** This group would audit the activities of the development organization, enforce quality standards, and ensure that processes are being followed and that no shortcuts are taken in the development cycle.
- **Documentation group.** A committee separate from the technical development group is needed to produce professional-quality user documentation and promote consistency across development projects and groups.

- **Configuration management.** Configuration managers are responsible for administering the source control tool, assigning file access privileges, satisfying build requests, and ensuring that the management of all software releases is controlled.
- **System test group.** Formalized product testing performed by a group separate from the group that implements the product helps to ensure product quality. This testing should occur during the development cycle and prior to delivery to a customer.
- **Beta coordinator.** The beta coordinator, a liaison between development and the rest of the company, works with customer service, field analysts, training, sales support, manufacturing, and other groups to impart product knowledge. As issues arise during the installation and beta cycle, the beta coordinator can help to resolve support issues that would otherwise consume valuable time for developers who could be fixing problems or moving on to other projects.

Successful IT organizations must not only adapt to the increasing pace of change in accordance with the logarithmic change in information technology, they must also adapt to the scarcity of resources and the migration of the information industry from an art to a engineering discipline. Companies need to look closely at what they do best and decide if they should insource or outsource their application development. Whatever the decision, the IT organization has—as always—a lot of change to absorb in the next five years.

11

Application Integration

Briggs T. Pille and Robert K. Antczak

In the early days of information systems, applications focused on specific functional areas or departmental needs. Financial systems, lab systems, and pharmacy systems were designed to service the individual user constituencies of the departments. When individuals required access to multiple systems, they often needed two separate terminals to gain access.

Trends in the healthcare industry created the continuum of care and the integrated delivery network, which have increased the need to access information across many facilities and locations. This need is one of the driving forces behind application integration, defined as the process of combining the information management value of multiple business applications. This combination can be achieved through the sharing of data, program logic, and/or presentation services.

In this chapter, we will identify some objectives and potential benefits of application integration, provide an overview of various approaches to integration, and offer advice on how to develop a strategy.

Benefits of Application Integration

The objectives and benefits of application integration vary widely in different organizations. In general, though, most organizations that undertake application integration projects want their efforts to:

- improve operations by synchronizing data and eliminating manual double entry and tape swapping
- deliver increased value through access to enterprise information (for example, a clinician's ability to access episodic information about a patient regardless of the setting of care for previous encounters)
- assist in the transformation of data into informative information by enabling enterprise information management techniques
- improve information access and ease of use for end users. This may improve user acceptance and help users take advantage of the resources available to them

- facilitate a reasonable level of "best of breed" that delivers better functionality to users while reducing operational costs related to management and maintenance
- decrease reliance on a single vendor whose modules or products may not offer state-of-the-market functionality
- minimize development time and effort related to integration
- support the redesign of operational processes through workflow automation and event-driven programming
- improve information management through the centralization and standardization of common data management tasks
- enforce organizational policies on security and confidentiality across all enterprise information sources
- distribute information tasks and processing while maintaining a uniform information model and management strategy.

Components of Application Integration

Historically, the most common form of application integration is interfacing. However, interfaces are only a part of application integration; other approaches and tools can deliver a greater degree of integration and more of the related benefits. *Understanding the range of integration options available is an important step toward developing an integration strategy.*

Gartner Group's three components of an application can be used to build a framework for classifying integration opportunities. The Gartner Group used these to discuss client/server systems, but they are relevant to all applications. The three logical components are:

- **Data management**—the application modules or tools used to control data and data functions. This component could consist of a relational database management system (RDBMS) and routines created within the RDBMS environment (i.e., stored procedures) to manage and maintain the data.
- **Program logic**—the application code, which defines the automated process to be completed. This component, theoretically, contains the clinical, administrative, and general business rules that dictate the system's function.
- **User presentation**—the application modules used to display information to the end user. This should not be confused with the actual operating system of the end user device (e.g., Windows 95 is not part of the user presentation component).

Another approach used in identifying integration opportunities is to evaluate information systems within technology layers. Each box in Figure 11.1 represents a set of enterprise technologies that require integration strategies and standardization within each layer. Integration strategies between layers are evaluated concurrently to ensure compatibility across the information system domain.

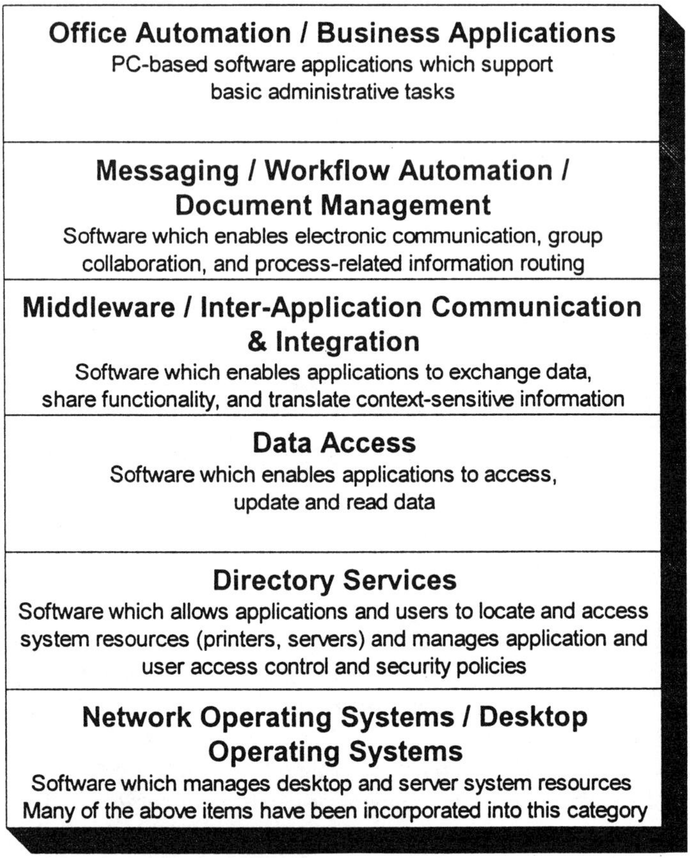

Layers of Enterprise Technology
Office Automation / Business Applications PC-based software applications which support basic administrative tasks
Messaging / Workflow Automation / Document Management Software which enables electronic communication, group collaboration, and process-related information routing
Middleware / Inter-Application Communication & Integration Software which enables applications to exchange data, share functionality, and translate context-sensitive information
Data Access Software which enables applications to access, update and read data
Directory Services Software which allows applications and users to locate and access system resources (printers, servers) and manages application and user access control and security policies
Network Operating Systems / Desktop Operating Systems Software which manages desktop and server system resources Many of the above items have been incorporated into this category

FIGURE 11.1. Layers of Enterprise Technology
© First Consulting Group 1998

In practice, a system implementation will contain portions of the components in Figure 11.2 across software objects, physical devices, and networks. Therefore, program logic may be found both in the database management system (e.g., as a stored procedure or trigger) and the end-user device (e.g., as event logic in a desktop application). Integration can focus on any one of these components, regardless of where they may reside. *The goals of the integration will determine the approach and components of focus.*

Stages of Application Integration

Application integration has evolved over time. Table 11.1 outlines the evolution of application integration in four stages.

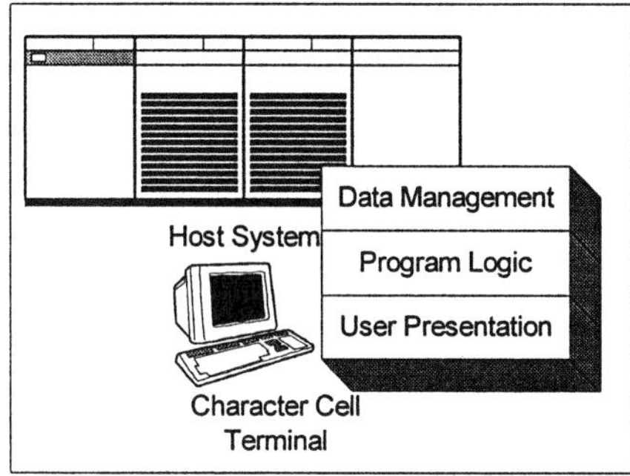

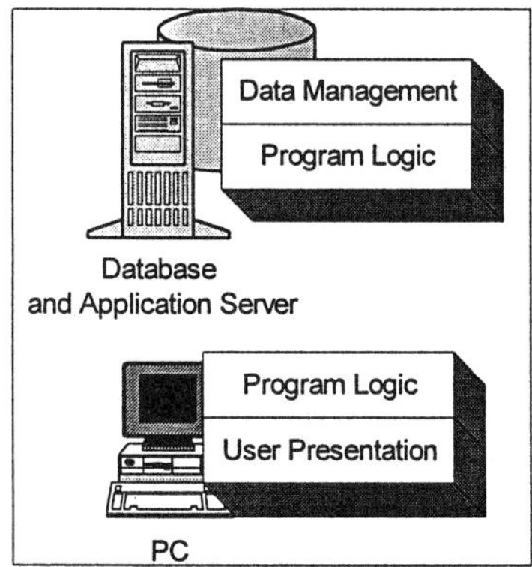

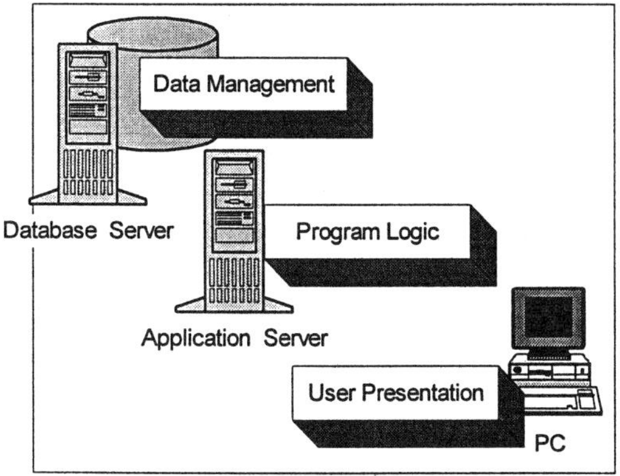

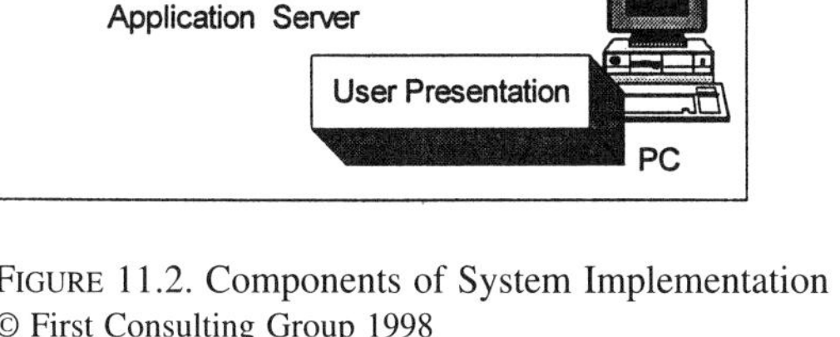

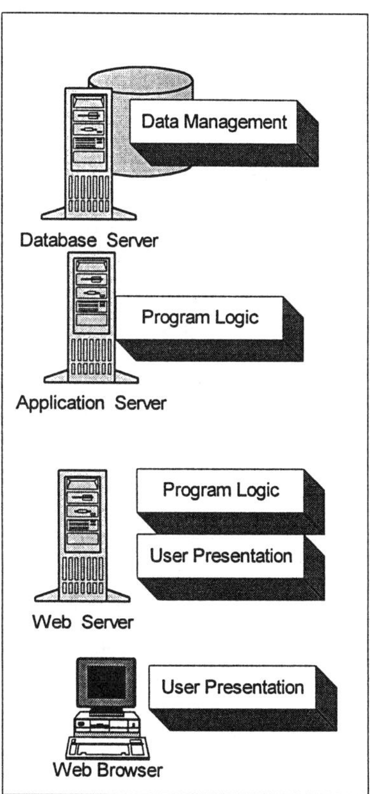

FIGURE 11.2. Components of System Implementation
© First Consulting Group 1998

TABLE 11.1. Stages of application integration.

Components	Stage 1	Stage 2	Stage 3	Stage 4
Data management	Data sharing	Data movement Data consolidation		Business components
Program logic			Rule consolidation	
User presentation	Multiple access		Universal client/ data access standards	

© First Consulting Group 1998

Stage 1 Integration

In the late 1980s and early 1990s, users were beginning to ask for access to more than one system, and they were not happy with multiple terminals. Stage 1 integration techniques tried to address this issue. The two solutions that emerged focused first on the user presentation component and then on data management.

- **Multiple access**—the use of a single end-user device to access multiple platforms and applications. This approach is characterized by "hot keying" between different application windows. In a heterogeneous (i.e., multiplatform) environment, an intelligent device (a personal computer) was required. Multiple access allowed a user to view or update information in multiple applications from a common user device. Besides freeing up the user's desktop space, it translated into incremental productivity gains.
- **Data sharing**—updating common data between systems via a point-to-point interface. An example of data sharing would be a point to point interface between an admission/discharge/transfer (ADT) system and a laboratory system to share patient demographics. Data sharing prevents the manual double keying of basic information.

Although Stage 1 integration techniques initially addressed the needs of the users, they left complex development and maintenance issues for ongoing operations. Stage 2 would attempt to solve these problems.

Stage 2 Integration

Stage 2 focused primarily on the data management components and attempted to address the operational issues Stage 1 had created. There were two major components to this stage:

- **Data movement**—using an application interface engine (AIE) to deliver a more standard means of accomplishing the benefits of data sharing. AIEs reduce interface development time and increase the level of standardization across interfaces. The market for AIEs exploded in the mid-1990s; examples include HUBLink, Datagate, and HCI Cloverleaf.
- **Data consolidation**—leveraging the power of an AIE to populate a data warehouse or repository (warehouses and repositories can play other roles in infor-

mation management; this chapter addresses only their role in application integration). Through the strong interfacing capabilities of an AIE, an organization can consolidate data into a common point of access. Data consolidation isolates operational systems from management query and reporting activity while permitting a greater manipulation of the data for management reporting purposes.

The industry impact of and market reaction to Stage 2 techniques were widespread. Hundreds of vendors came to market with an AIE and/or warehouse/repository solution. This second stage of application integration capability is a major enabler in the creation of an information management approach. Today, most healthcare organizations have implemented or are implementing Stage 2 techniques.

Stage 3 Integration

Stage 3 integration goes beyond the data management component to deliver additional value to an organization. Approaches in this stage leverage two key technology trends: Internet-based technology, and knowledge base and rule syntax standards. Although knowledge stores have not impacted information systems development as strongly as Internet technology has, standards for clinical and administrative rule creation and maintenance have allowed some organizations to share common program logic across disparate systems. Arden syntax and drug interaction knowledge stores are examples of this technology.

Three approaches comprise this third stage of integration. While these approaches are independent of one another, they may be most valuable if implemented together.

Universal Client

This refers to the use of a common client interface program to access all applications. The universal client promises to deliver true user transparency. The user would not know what application was being used or what database was being queried. A universal client would reduce end-user training requirements and create a seamless view of enterprise information management. If an integrated view of information from multiple information sources is deemed beneficial, then the ability of a universal client technology to streamline business and clinical processes also should be viewed as vital.

The universal client's greatest value lies in its potential to provide access to core clinical processes to new groups of users. The ability of patients to actively participate in information systems designed to support their access to care is one example of the universal client's potential. Today, web browsers and Internet technology are providing a potential means of attaining a universal client. Although a subset of Internet standards have been adopted by the information systems industry, many barriers still exist in integrating Internet-compliant systems. Vendors exploit features not addressed by the standards in order to differentiate their products. Security and data integrity are major concerns with a client integration–based approach. We discuss recent approaches to universal client deployment next.

Data Access Standards

Along with the universal client, data access methods such as open data base connectivity (ODBC), Java database connectivity (JDBC), and data access objects (DAO) standards are allowing personal computer (PC) and web-based applications access to disparate data stores without requiring complex data consolidation and data movement. Merging organizations can benefit from the ease of implementing data access standards, but may later need to address performance and scalability issues.

Rule Consolidation

This is simply an extension of data consolidation techniques, although the theory of storing program logic in a central location can be extended to formularies related to clinical and administrative subjects. The complexities of payer and provider reimbursement policies and clinical rules notwithstanding, many systems have leveraged drug-drug and drug-allergy interactions across disparate systems. The ability to create and maintain rules that map to an organization's processes will increase overall information and organization flexibility. An organization's evaluating integration strategies must consider how business and clinical rules will be stored, modified, and extended. Process modeling techniques provide an opportunity for information systems to store workflow rules in easily extensible forms. Rather than codifying operational processes within rigid, complex, and hidden program code, organizations must endeavor to reflect processes in data stores and implementation-independent formats. An applications state and branch logic should be stored in database tables along with the traditional data elements. Some leading-edge healthcare organizations are investigating and even implementing Stage 3 solutions, but the majority is only now learning of the techniques. Other information-intensive industries (e.g., financial services) are embracing the emerging Stage 3 techniques.

Stage 4 Integration

The final stage of integration focuses on business components—for example, the use of object technology and development techniques to share program logic and data management between applications. There are many potential benefits to promoting object orientation, but one of the greatest is inherent application integration. By containing a subset of common functionality, a business component can be accessed by many applications. In order for this potential to be realized, however, industry organizations like the Andover Working Group and the Object Management Group must overcome integration barriers between object models and directory schemes.

As Stage 3 and 4 integration approaches continue to evolve, vendors are defining often competing standards for application integration within each of the system components. The few healthcare organizations pursuing this level of integration are balancing the benefits of the technology with the risks of early adoption. The risks include teaming with a vendor that may not deliver or choosing a standard that may not survive.

User presentation solutions are focusing on the extension of web-browser technology. These extensions may enable the integration of office automation and messaging applications with clinical and administrative systems. However, the use of a particular vendor's technology may preclude the information management benefits to be gained by a higher degree of integration. The prevalence of Microsoft Windows technology is driving the adoption of the distributed component object model (DCOM). As a result, user organizations may be limiting the potential benefits of a universal client solution, since not all system vendors or business affiliates are adhering to this approach.

Applet and object model solutions like ActiveX/Java and Java Bean/DCOM allow the integration of applications, both at centrally controlled server devices and at the end-user device. Components can share exposed data and functionality when following rules enforced by a particular object model. An object request broker typically accomplishes enforcement of rules and security across a network.

Another approach allows applications to pass data between them within the context of a user session. Although such an approach does not eliminate the need for object request broker technology, it does simplify some integration efforts. For example, proposals by the Clinical Context Object Workgroup provide developers with facilities to pass clinical data patient demographics to other applications running on the user's workstation. We emphasize, however, that *enforcement of security and organizational policies across information systems will not be realized until formal business object standards and protocols are adopted.*

Defining an Application Integration Strategy

Before it can achieve the full potential of performance improvements associated with these techniques, an organization must define an application integration strategy. Stage 1 approaches could be defined on an application-by-application basis, but to effectively utilize Stages 2 through 4 techniques, an overall application integration strategy must be in place. An application integration strategy is an essential component of an application architecture.

The first step is to define an organization's information model. This model defines objects and relationships between objects and allows application integration to occur within the context of recognized business entities and functions.

The second step is to decide where the most benefit can be realized through integration. This step must be closely linked to an organization's overall information management strategy. Any or all of the logical application components can be the focus of integration.

The third step is to decide upon the tools and combination of tools to accomplish the integration. Is a universal client access approach to disparate systems more cost-effective and efficient than data consolidation? The answer to this question must be based on organization-specific integration goals.

An application integration strategy should be implemented over a reasonable time frame. A 12- to 18-month migration window may be required to accomplish the defined strategy. Appropriate prioritization of systems, interfaces, and user constituencies will help an organization deliver significant value during a phased migration. When planning for implementation, organizations should also consider the potential need to utilize Stage 2 and 3 technologies (establishing an integration baseline) prior to attempting Stage 4 integration solutions.

Conclusions

Clearly, application integration can play a significant role in information management. In fact, we believe application integration is required to perform information management in a heterogeneous environment.

Application integration techniques have evolved to deliver significant benefits. As this chapter has indicated, the various stages of integration provide different benefits and require a different level of implementation effort. An organization must establish application integration goals before selecting what technologies, solutions, and products are appropriate for its environment. We believe evolving techniques like the ones suggested in this chapter can provide opportunities for performance improvement through more comprehensive sharing of data and increased operational efficiency, delivered through program logic and user presentation-based integration.

12

Technical Infrastructure: Power for the Enterprise

David Dimond, Michael Gorsage, Joseph Casper, and Judith V. Douglas

The evolution of the healthcare marketplace imposes new demands on the use of information technology. Strategies for process redesign and operational effectiveness hold the key to surviving and gaining competitive advantage. The underlying information technology architecture—the technical infrastructure—must be flexible enough to adapt to the changing demands of the healthcare industry, and structured to be both cost effective and manageable.

Networking technologies are an essential part of an information systems infrastructure—but only a part. Deficiencies or incompatibilities in the infrastructure may limit the organization's ability to support business requirements and mitigate nonconforming technologies. Because these limitations can be pervasive, infrastructure issues merit the highest level of attention throughout the enterprise. Filling in the "gaps" in technical infrastructure is the prerequisite for plugging personal computers, telephones, and video conferencing devices into the "communications outlet"—the outlet that enables end users to access information, participate in core processes, and enter into collaborative activities.

Defining Technical Infrastructure

Technical infrastructure (TI) can be difficult to understand. It's more than the network—but what is it? We look to the term itself for clarification. As infrastructure, it is literally underneath or below and out of sight, and it is technical, with multiple components.

Like electricity, TI empowers and enables. The communications outlet in the wall gives access to a host of applications on servers, files on storage devices, and real-time collaboration with individuals via video or voice—down the hall or miles away at enterprise headquarters. The source of the connection is irrelevant as demand for information and collaboration power keeps coming.

Like electricity, with its transformers, power lines, wiring, switches, and end-user appliances, TI consists of multiple components. The cable plant within a given facility provides the physical infrastructure, including wiring closets. Network electronics support data communications, both on local area and wide area networks (LANs/WANs). Often sharing lines with data communications are voice systems, including in-house telephone systems called private branch exchanges (PBXs), with access to local and long-distance services, and value-added networks. The TI's end-user appliances are typically telephone stations and desktop personal computers linked to a variety of enterprise or remote services.

Planning for Demand

The tendency is to take TI, like electricity, for granted. We don't stop to consider that almost everything depends on it. When infrastructure fails, we find ourselves in the same situation as when the electricity goes off, and we turn on the water and the pump doesn't work or we adjust the thermostat on the gas furnace and the blower doesn't kick in. When the power's on, we forget these electrical components exist, and we can't say how many switch plates and outlets we have. When the power is off, normal activities stop and we go in search of the switch box.

The same is true for technical infrastructure. Call centers, data repositories, applications—they all depend on TI. When the TI fails, information ceases to flow, and the enterprise loses power. When the system is down, admitting clerks can not validate a patient's information without pulling or creating paper backup. At best the result is slow service and decreased customer satisfaction, much the same as when the system is "just slow today." Of course, in health care, slow response time and the lack of information can have much more serious consequences. For caregivers, administrators, customer service agents and other end users, TI problems can impair the ability to perform their job functions, decreasing their productivity.

We stress that TI "failure" occurs in different forms. It can mean total stoppage, not unheard of but fortunately not common. Or it can have "limited impact," as when all functions dependent upon a particular server are affected. *As technology becomes more sophisticated and enterprises become more complex, we are seeing more subtle manifestations of TI failure.* As an example, we cite cases in which the existing TI lacks the bandwidth required to deliver new applications and information between locations. In some cases, the connection may be there, the power is still on, but the end user is experiencing a "brownout" or a degraded level of service. Often the degraded level of service will force the application to time out and break the connection, much as circuit breakers are flipped when demands exceed the availability of electrical current. Here, the TI fails in that it limits the effectiveness and benefits of continuing investments in information systems and collaborative processes. The TI also fails if it constrains the efforts of skilled (and expensive!) technical staff to develop and deploy flexible, scaleable information systems.

Power Industry Model

The electrical utility industry commonly overprovisions the capacity of delivery systems. This practice ensures that systems can handle future demands—the unplanned neighborhoods and commercial structures that may be built in a given community sometime in the future. Even on a daily basis, electrical utilities proactively generate excess power that can be delivered on demand. Their only planning mechanism is the level of service (the amount of amperage or amps) that has been provisioned to homes and buildings on the electrical grid. Brownouts occur only when extreme weather conditions create anomalies in power consumption. Demand-side management programs (energy-efficient lighting, water heater blankets) help consumers use power more efficiently, minimizing and leveling out consumption requirements.

The power industry also has strict standards for capacity planning, infrastructure provisioning, power service levels, delivery specifications, and line termination. This enables the consumer to procure, plug, and power commodities. This also allows the utility to develop a pool of employees with a commodity level of skill for proactively managing and reactively repairing the electrical delivery system. Standards create an environment that gives electricians the ability to work confidently anywhere in the United States and for utilities to borrow linepersons during service outages in extreme weather conditions. Similarly, a standard-based TI allows health plan and care delivery organizations to procure contract resources during peak project needs and positions them favorably for outsourcing portions of the TI.

Today many healthcare enterprises are still debating whether to manage or "overprovision" resources in their standards-based enterprise networks. It is time, we believe, to choose the latter option. We should model TI—the information source—on the utility industry. Our voice and data network engineers should handle capacity needs, provision service levels, and measure demands by proactively testing applications requirements and doing trend analysis on an ongoing basis.

We are convinced that planning for excess capacity and demand is the only realistic approach. Development of the components needed to implement high-capacity TI is continuing. Moore's Law—the number of transistors that can be placed on microchip doubles every 18 months—has proved true to date, and Intel's Andy Grove expects it to hold up for 10 more years, given current technical knowledge. According to its corollary Internet Law, the data-transmission capacity demands of consumers double every three to four months, necessitating an annual growth factor of 10. Clearly, technology places demands on planners, implementors, and users alike.

The Business Case

The principal purpose of investing in [information technology] is not overhead cost reduction but value-creation. . . . The objective of all investments is to improve overall organizational performance. (Strassmann 1997, p. 19).

Implementing a TI enables the healthcare enterprise to respond to business drivers integral to its mission. *The net effect of TI implementation is to make the enterprise light on its feet, able to respond quickly and proactively, and to man-*

age mission-critical information and processes. It provides the power and the ways to hook up to and deliver that power quickly, without major retrofitting and customizing. With the rapid pace of technology development and replacement, the so-called "Gates factor," the ability to deploy and to upgrade is critical.

Approaching any TI implementation, we stress there are certain guiding principles:

- Offer universal connectivity to all internal and external information resources (access will be provided only where appropriate).
- Support a common set of devices, applications, and tools for all authorized users.
- Integrate information flows across the enterprise.
- Design reliability and availability to meet business needs.
- Provide flexibility to adapt to continually changing business requirements and technology developments.
- Abstract TI for applications and information to support "point-of-need" delivery throughout the enterprise.
- Architect solutions that minimize future capital investment and operations expenses.
- Standardize on TI hardware and software vendors and deployment procedures across the enterprise.
- Provide "views of information" based on user needs and profiles.

Following these principles helps ensure that the TI being implemented does in fact deliver benefits to the healthcare enterprise, as shown in Table 12.1.

Technical infrastructure enables disparate systems and collaborative processes to be rapidly enabled in a manner that ensures they are widely accessible yet secure, easily integrated, and operated with sufficient and consistent levels of service. Simply stated, *TI provides agility.*

The ongoing advances in open-system technology standards make these benefits possible by improving interoperability and supporting functionality and overall flexibility with a consistent TI. The extent to which benefits are realized

TABLE 12.1. Benefits of technical infrastructure.

Benefits of technical infrastructure	
• Technology positioned to support a majority of information requirements	• Proactive ability to respond to changing technology needs in the healthcare industry
• Orderly migration to new technologies	• Faster deployment of critical applications
• Reduction of idle equipment	• Consistent configuration and implementation
• Ability to rapidly provide network services	• Greater efficiency of information retrieval
• Higher utilization of information systems	• Consistent and cost-effective information security
• Improved portability of applications and components	• Ease of network management and network troubleshooting

© First Consulting Group 1998

is directly related to the extent to which the architecture is implemented across the entire enterprise. Deviations from the design reduce the benefits that the TI can offer.

This relationship becomes evident when we look at some of the key requirements within integrated delivery networks (IDNs). Messaging, patient scheduling, and flow coordination—all must be enterprise-wide to deliver full benefits. In like manner, data access and data integration are enterprise-wide needs, in the full range of acute and ambulatory settings. Increasingly, with the emphasis on outcomes and performance measurement, data integration reaches across both clinical and financial systems. The TI has to be robust to support these needs and the growing numbers of client/server or web-enabled applications and intelligent desktop workstations across the enterprise. These growth areas underscore the importance of flexibility and specially tailored views across the continuum of care.

The costs of implementing and upgrading the TI can be high, but so are the costs associated with not doing so. In the case of networking (again, only part of the TI but definitely a hot topic for newly formed IDNs), an inconsistent, nonconforming approach can entail additional hardware, retraining, specialization, increased hardware/software maintenance costs, custom development efforts, and the loss of economies of scale. Although these costs can be difficult to document, experience demonstrates that organizations without networking standards and guidelines realize increases in capital and operational costs. Standardization doesn't inhibit flexibility—it maximizes interoperability between network and computer systems. This, in turn, increases the value of the TI and the information system it supports.

Architectural Planning for TI

When the intent is to provide integrated services across the continuum of care, business strategy demands an enterprise network, including cabling and network infrastructure, to support the information needs and requirements of its multiple facilities. Within this context, TI architectural planning becomes a critical initial and ongoing function, and the TI architecture becomes a reference manual for network planners, implementers, department heads, executives, technology partners, and end users. It includes as its base an accurate assessment of the current environment and a precise identification of requirements.

The TI architectural plan defines how to convert business strategies into a technical network infrastructure that can support world-class clinical, financial, and administration systems. The plan provides the blueprints that guide choices regarding network systems and services as well as implementation activities over the next three to five years. As shown in Table 12.2, technology focus areas include connectivity, accessibility, functionality, and manageability.

Sections within the plan address these four network technology focus areas. The section on design provides conceptual models of how all the network com-

TABLE 12.2. Network technology focus area.

Focus area	Objective	Component examples
Network connectivity	Provide the physical network infrastructure that links all network and telephony station interfaces	Structured cabling systems, network electronics, WAN systems, PBX systems, transport and interconnection protocols
Network accessibility	Provide the hardware and/or software that enable(s) end-user access to systems and services	Network interface cards and protocols, directory services, single sign-on technologies
Network functionality	Provide the applications and services that integrate and present information	Network and desktop operation systems, electronic mail, all other shared applications and devices
Network manageability	Provide the services and components that enable network and systems management	Help desk, component intelligence, network component element managers

© First Consulting Group 1998

ponents fit together. The standards and guidelines section identifies technical standards, itemizes services and products where appropriate, and includes project plans for implementing the models.

All network designs are derived from the TI architectural plan. Strategic in nature, the planning document provides the framework and the methodology for migrating from existing systems to a network that can support current and future business strategies. A 30,000-foot view of where the healthcare enterprise is heading, the plan directs the next phase, network design.

The network design phase identifies specific projects needed to meet specific business requirements. Tactical in nature, network design examines what specifically needs to be done in order to migrate from existing systems to an enterprise-wide network supporting current and future business strategies. This "sea-level" approach identifies projects based on recommendations from the network architecture and details engineering specifications for each task. Grounded in technology life cycle methodology, this approach requires continuous updates to optimize flexibility. The product of this phase is the network design document that will drive selection and implementation.

A typical network design project takes from two to four months to complete, depending upon a number of factors:

- complexity of the network environment (number of networking schemes, protocols, PBXs, devices, etc.)
- types of network traffic (data, voice, images, video, etc.) and future bandwidth requirements
- size of the organization (users, sites, etc.)
- types of application requirements and business processes impacted by the effort

- number of hardware and software platforms
- number of different geographic locations
- experience of internal resources
- desirability of bringing in consultants
- knowledge of the environment.

Network Design

The first step in the network design process is project identification; this constitutes from 5 to 15 percent of the total design process. Tasks here include reviewing the network architecture; confirming business drivers, network requirements, and technology assessments; and investigating current migration strategies. The output is a list of projects for each component of the network framework. The precision of the TI architectural plan, cooperation of client personnel, and validity of project assumptions are all factors in the success of this step.

Next comes gap analysis, also claiming from 5 to 15 percent of the overall effort. Focusing on the differences between what exists and what is recommended in the TI plan, this step reviews design areas, confirms whether or not they are addressed, and revisits project assumptions. The intent here is to detail what needs to be done in order to migrate from existing systems to a network supporting current and future business strategies. Although this step does not entail a high level of effort, it does demand a high level of judgment and expertise. Understanding of network and application requirements in the current environment must be matched by insights into the network architecture requirements set forth in the TI plan.

The third step, estimated at 45 to 55 percent of total effort, is the most time-consuming. When completed, it provides a comprehensive draft network design document and an engineering specification package for each individual project, as shown in Table 12.3. Each package includes task lists, product comparisons, a bill of materials, diagrams, and any other supporting documentation required. Accurate and current vendor information, not always easy to obtain, is critical here.

The fourth and final step in the network design process is development of a high-level integrated project work plan. Set at 25 percent of effort, this uses the draft design document to produce an overall project schedule plan, including timelines and workflow. Tasks here include identifying all projects, priorities between projects, dependencies between projects, and resources available for each project. The outputs for this last step include the final network design document and engineering specification packages, along with the network design migration plan and the integrated work plan. At a minimum, this work plan should cover a two-year time period and result in completing the network requirements set forth in the TI architectural plan.

TABLE 12.3. Areas/tools requiring engineering specification packages.

Network component area	Function	Example of associated tools
Physical infrastructure	Provide physical connectivity between data and voice devices on the enterprise network	Backbone and device wiring, hubs, routers, switches, network interface cards (NICs)
LAN technologies	Allow user groups bound by geography and/or function to share and leverage common resources	Backbone and workgroup network schemes and protocols, ethernet, asynchronous transfer mode, Intranets
WAN technologies	Provide connectivity for disparate systems and organizations over geographically dispersed areas	Protocols, services, ATM, frame relay, leased lines, Internet connections, Extranets
Remote access technologies	Support communications for remote users	Dial-up network access, LAN-to-remote host, remote user-to-LAN host, virtual private networks
Network services	Facilitate transfer, storage, and retrieval of information within a networked environment	Network operating systems, file sharing services, print services, backup, directory services, voice services
Network applications	Facilitate the operation of network-dependent applications, including standard and advanced voice communications services	Office automation, e-mail, groupware, imaging, videoconferencing, Internet/Intranet, interactive voice response, computer telephony integration, automatic call distributors, multipoint conferencing/control units (MCU)
Telephony services	Provide point-to-point and multipoint collaboration via voice communications	PBXs, conference bridges, transport services, value-added networks
End-user devices	Provide the interface between network resources and end user	Terminals, personal computers, desktop operating systems, telephones, graphical user interfaces
Management systems and services	Facilitate the monitoring, control, and administration of the enterprise network	Network management systems, consoles and probes, network sniffers, trend analysis tools and correlation engines, call management systems, traffic manage systems, simulation tools

© First Consulting Group 1998

A New TI Philosophy

Managing

Traditionally, implementation follows design, and operations support follows implementation. In the accelerated environment of network planning, this is still true, albeit in a somewhat limited sense. Postdesign tasks still include the procurement of equipment, installation planning, integration testing, acceptance testing, policy and procedure development, and end-user and support training. Postimplementation activities still involve maintaining and supporting the network technology. However, given the growth factor and the varied lifespans for different technologies, operational tasks like performance tracking, benefits analysis, and network security auditing must become part of a feedback loop. Only if they do can the TI continue to offer the flexibility the enterprise requires.

Staffing and Outsourcing

Like other industries, from financial services to computer vendors, healthcare enterprises are finding it increasingly difficult to recruit and retain skilled technical staff. At the 1998 meeting of the Health Information Management and Systems Society (HIMSS), attendees ranked staffing as their top concern on the annual leadership survey. The fact is, individuals who are technically competent in state-of-the-art technologies are precious resources, expensive to obtain and to keep.

For this reason, there is new discussion of outsourcing. We believe that outsourcing may offer solutions in some instances, but a decision regarding any capability central to the core mission of an organization cannot be taken lightly.

The Challenge

Technical issues can be addressed. It is the human issues—organizational politics and funding, workflow and process design, professional development and training—that persist. These issues impact TI and are impacted by it. Certainly networking must remain in the control of the enterprise, outsourced or not.

With top-level attention to TI, the enterprise will attain new agility and become capable of meeting the challenges it faces. *Power to the enterprise!*

Reference

Strassmann, P.A. 1997. *The Squandered Computer: Evaluating the Business Alignment of Information Technologies.* New Canaan, Conn.: Information Economics Press.

13

Emerging Technologies

GORDON HEINRICH AND GAIL HINTE

As new technologies emerge, health care works to make use of the capabilities they offer. Intranets, the Internet, and the World Wide Web support an increasingly robust communications environment. Wireless and portable technologies are providing access at the point of care. Clearly, technical innovations continue to keep pace with and support the evolution of health care. We see incredible opportunities for synergy between these two industries, each of which is changing at an astounding rate.

To illustrate this potential, we have chosen to focus on two distinctly different technologies. One helps build relationships between healthcare organizations and their external customers. The other facilitates information flow within the organization and supports the move toward the computerized patient record. Both technologies—call centers and document management—can be categorized as "emerging" in that they are just beginning to impact health care. Both serve "customers," one outside the organization, the other inside. Each functions optimally when it becomes part of an enterprise information architecture, not a stand-alone tool. We believe the focus on customer service as a key part of business strategy is what drives the decisions to adopt these technologies, and the alignment between technical capabilities and operational effectiveness is what distinguishes the new role of information management in health care.

Call Centers

Hello, how may I help you?

In today's market, call centers are a critical component in a customer service strategy that builds long-lasting relationships and ultimately contributes to the market share and the bottom line. "The business of business," Peter Drucker wrote in 1979, "is getting and keeping customers." Embracing a customer service focus will go miles in keeping customers happy and yours. According to a survey on why customers quit, 68 percent of those who leave a supplier do so because of perceived indifference on the part of the owner, manager, or some employee (Le Doeuf 1987). A comprehensive strategy is required, detailing how to communicate and interact with customers. *Customers want to communicate any time, any way, and about anything.* They want to call, e-mail, fax, and browse to obtain services, complain, and provide feedback. We believe implementing a call center as the "front line" provides the best method for handling all forms of communications.

Build Long-Lasting Relationships

Relationships are based on mutual trust and common understanding. To build relationships, the organization has to make it easy to interact or do business. Today's healthcare marketplace is full of highly complex organizations with "add as you grow" customer interactions. It is hard for customers to navigate the system if they know their way around and almost impossible if they don't. It is difficult to make an appointment, pay a bill, or get information about a procedure. A call center can provide the leverage to simplify the customer interface for the full range of communications, from telephone interactions to automated services, fax services, and e-mail.

In building the relationship, start by delighting the customers. Understand their needs. What is their expectation of service? Is it different for different people? Because we think it is, we recommend segmenting the population to address cultural and demographic preferences including languages and technology adoption. Consider the service from start to finish, in what we call the interaction strategy. Remember that any point along the way offers the opportunity to build the relationship—or destroy it. The first step in the process is usually the phone call, making an excellent interaction especially important.

What constitutes an excellent interaction? Let's consider the customer who wants to book an appointment. The number should be easy to find, the phone should be answered promptly, and the agent who handles the call should be pleasant and knowledgeable enough to fill the customer's request. Note what this entails: simplifying the phone numbers, staffing the call center with enough good agents, and providing the tools and information those agents need.

Customer expectations of call centers tend to run high. Many have used 800 numbers in other industries that have invested heavily to define excellent service. According to a survey by the Center for Customer-Driven Quality at Purdue University, the goal of most companies is to have an average speed of answer under 20 seconds. *We believe that customers expect healthcare organizations to meet the standards set by the collective universe of call centers.*

The lifetime value of a customer is often debated and varies by industry. One fact is clear, however: the average business spends six times more to attract new customers than to keep old ones (Le Doeuf 1987). It makes sense to invest capital where it has the greatest impact, and the call center provides controls and mechanisms to build and maintain customer relationships. Although some organizations view the call center as a cost reduction opportunity, we see it as a strategic business imperative.

Invest in Appropriate Technologies

Although it has been available for years, call center technology is currently in an innovation cycle and changing rapidly. Deciding which technologies to deploy can be difficult. Service strategy, technology architecture, and cost effectiveness are key. To accomplish the goals of the strategy, the technology should be sophisticated enough to offer an easy-to-use system to the customer. To fit into the overall enterprise architecture, the technology should conform to standards where appropriate and provide management tools for easy support and maintenance. Because call centers concentrate traffic into relatively few locations, a highly robust infrastructure is essential. In addition, remember that the cost of solutions varies greatly. Matching functionality with cost helps to achieve maximum impact for money spent.

There are many issues to deal with when designing and architecting a call center solution. The system must be designed for a high volume of transactions, mixed media, real-time interactions, and mission-critical services. It must also be simple to use, manage, and maintain. Luckily, call center vendors have invested aggressively in this market and have innovated extensively, creating different approaches and many options.

Call center technology includes a number of components: automatic call distributors (ACDs), private branch exchanges (PBXs), 800 networks and private voice networks, local and wide area networks (LAN/WANs), host access, agent applications, desktop computers, and servers. Computer telephony integration (CTI) links these components. In effect, CTI is the glue that makes a fully integrated call center a reality.

Today's call centers are "intelligent" as well as integrated. They make it possible to manage calls, routing them to the appropriate agent who has the needed information right on the desktop. This information can be stored in a number of ways. The intelligence can be located on the public network, the ACD network, or within the call center. Routing choice, member interaction, reporting, and voice and data synchronization can happen at any level. The decision on where to perform the action should factor in the installed base of equipment, the amount of sophistication required, the cost basis involved, and the degree of risk considered acceptable.

Prepare to Manage Mixed Environments

As interactions become increasingly electronic, overall interaction strategies have even greater impact. Customers want to communicate how and when they choose, using a combination of telephone, e-mail, web, fax, and video. Call centers must be ready to address the various mixed media that customers will use. To prepare for the inevitable, the technology used to create the call center must be flexible, cost effective, and a good fit with the overall enterprise.

Call centers also have met the web. First, a "call me" button was incorporated on a web page, integrating the Internet with the call center. This can have a big impact on interaction strategies and operations. Next came pushing web pages to the caller, using them to explain complex information in a rich environment. Today's web technology is being used within the four walls of the call center. Intranet technology provides critical information via web-enabled applications. Thanks to a very quick development cycle, web applications can be up and running in a short time and modified quickly to accommodate rapid consumer changes.

Today's sophisticated ACDs can route calls based on skills or dynamically based on the status of the system. Calls can be routed to the last agent to speak with the caller or to the best agent for the job. This personalizes the interaction, helping to build relationships with members while still realizing the cost advantage. As ACDs become more "open," they can accept third-party enhancements, routing and reporting software, load balancing, and more. Design of equipment strategies can emphasize the intelligence, the public network, ACDs, or third-party middleware.

As always, change has its downside. As the call center opens up to more than just voice, agents must deal with an increasing amount of complexity. Mixed media calls—e-mail, web-enabled, and video—require agents to make use of sophisticated routing and advanced tools. Managing more than voice calls has an impact on how the call center operates and what type of systems it needs to deal in this mixed environment.

Interactive Voice Response

Today's customers use interactive voice response (IVR) systems for a variety of purposes, from banking to refilling prescriptions and more. It gives customers access 24 hours a day, 7 days a week—a real convenience for busy people who want to get things done. In addition, it can off-load routine interactions and free up agents to handle more complicated queries.

If designed correctly, IVR can be a valuable tool. Take menus, for example. As the customer interface for this technology, they should reflect accurately the customer interaction strategy (CIS). They should be easy to use and written from the caller's point of view. To give real value, they should perform important tasks.

We all know how frustrating poorly designed IVR systems can be. In a survey of 409 IVR applications across multiple industries reported at a 1997 conference on computer telephony, the Enterprise Integration Group, Inc., identified the following main problem areas:

- Lack of customer-oriented design
- Poor menu construction and testing
- Excessive application complexity
- Lack of standard navigation keys

Fortunately, these problems can be fixed. A good design strategy that addresses human factors and includes usability testing will go a long way to improve customer service. In turn, customer satisfaction will help increase penetration of IVRs and off-load traffic from the call center's agent pool.

IVRs are useful because *almost* everyone has a telephone. Still, the 12-button interface is limiting. We should look to other emerging technologies—speech recognition and natural language interface. With them, a user can talk in continuous, natural speech with the IVR prompting to catch missed phrases.

Call Me

As the Web is integrated into the call center, the use of "call me" buttons is taking off. The web page user can push the button to connect with or get a call back from a call center agent. The agent can look at the same web page as the user and help the user navigate through the page. This is very effective in dealing with complicated information such as open enrollment options.

"Call me" buttons, however, are no excuse for poorly designed web pages. Web pages should always be designed within the CIS and conform to good design and usability principles. If users do not find the page usable, they will hit the "call me" button and the call center agent will have to deal with a complex situation.

Workflow

Workflow software is rapidly finding its way into the call center. It allows a transaction to be traced from the initial encounter all the way to the end and archived for future reference or reporting. To provide the maximum advantage and flexibility, workflow applications must be integrated into the CTI and networking fabric. Once the enterprise is integrated with the call center, workflow software can help establish optimal relationships with customers.

Reporting

Once a call center is up and running, reporting becomes critical to its success. The technology provides many routine reports, including those on ACDs, PBXs, networks, applications, and IVR.

However, to make a call center easy to manage and to understand its impact on operations, the data must be combined with business data to produce meaningful reports. Designing an effective data warehousing strategy and methods to mine the data is essential to getting the most out of any call center.

Keep Focused

There is an abundance of call center technology available on the market today, making it possible to build all sorts of interesting solutions. Even so, it is not easy to architect, design, and implement a system that is flexible and robust. Customers, after all, are an ever-changing, mission-critical, strategically important asset—and understanding how customers want to communicate and interact with the enterprise is critical. *With so many options available, there is one ruling principle: Use the technology to make things simple.*

Document Management

Call centers are out in the open, so most of us are familiar with what they can do. Document management, on the other hand, remains behind the scenes and a bit of a mystery. Critics consider it a stopgap measure to allow simultaneous access to the paper-based patient record—which will soon be obsolete—and to reduce costs by eliminating microfilming.

Despite our industry's misunderstanding of the capabilities and benefits of document management, we believe reality favors those who implement this technology in health care. Why would document management be used in banks and insurance companies worldwide, but not be applicable to health care? Why would American Express embrace the technology as a benefit to operations, while healthcare organizations dismiss it as nearly obsolete?

Components of Document Management

It is easy to confuse document management with the simplest form of imaging technology—scanning. Scanners convert paper documents to electronic media; records are then individually indexed for future retrieval and stored using optical disks. Indexing is done using an admission/discharge/transfer (ADT) interface for basic demographics, augmented with either optical character recognition (OCR) or bar coding for document identification (e.g., consent for treatment form). This process can be time-consuming and resource-intensive, especially with the massive amounts of paper generated by healthcare organizations, but it will continue to be essential for inputting nonautomated and handwritten forms, such as physician notes.

Scanning, however, is just one form of input for document management systems. It is supplemented by computer output to laser disk (COLD) technology, for forms and data that are already automated, like lab results, face sheets, and transcribed notes. This electronic transmission and indexing of information bypasses the scanning and indexing processes required by paper files. Both scanned and COLD images are stored initially on magnetic media for immediate retrieval (less than three seconds) and are permanently housed in jukeboxes that manage multiple optical disks. The process is deceptively simple, however. Document input using multiple technologies still requires human intervention—something to remember when implementing document management.

Imaging software, relational databases, and software applications allow the document management system to store, cross-index, retrieve, and perform studies on images and related indices. Chart completion and electronic signature software facilitates physician and clinician online use from any image-enabled workstation within the hospital network. The security of patient data is enhanced by limiting access to document and patient types on a need-to-know basis and by creating audit trails of any viewed documents.

Benefits of Document Management

The imaging component in particular can offer immediate benefits:

- **Space savings.** One jukebox is equivalent to a fileroom of medical records.
- **Simultaneous access to the same record.** Contention for records is eliminated.
- **Immediate access to the record.** "Calling down for records" becomes an obsolete function.
- **No lost records.** Once imaged into the system, records are always available with proper authorization.
- **Disaster recovery.** Electronic file backups stored off-site eliminate the dangers of file room disasters, typically impossible to recover.
- **No microfilm.** Optical disk storage eliminates costs associated with microfilming and provides better-quality copies.

Real as they are, these benefits merely scratch the surface. The pivotal benefits of document management technology are often overlooked: clinical data repository (CDR) enhancement, medical records automation, and enterprise-wide workflow development.

Clinical Data Repository Enhancement

Designed to collect patient care information and display it in user-friendly format, CDRs support improvements in patient care (immediate access to patient information), operational efficiencies (avoid duplicate testing), risk management (online drug-drug/food interactions), and managed care compliance (available drug formularies). We have no doubt that organizations should be encouraged to continue CDR development, especially if physicians will be the primary users of the system.

However, the CDR can be populated with electronic data only, and the resulting limitations constitute a serious problem for organizations with minimal medical record automation. Document management integrated with the CDR can make the full patient record available to clinicians, by including past history, transfer records, and other documents imaged into the system. As organizations become more automated, scanned images are replaced with electronic data, but they are still required for those areas where automation may be implemented more slowly (e.g., physician progress notes) or perhaps not at all (e.g., transfer records).

Table 13.1 shows which kind of system—data repository or document management—works best with various types of patient care.

TABLE 13.1. Data repositories versus document management.

	System type	
Activity to support patient care	Data repository	Document management
Access to current patient care records	√	√
Handwritten notes, tracings, and patient consent forms		√
Old, extra-enterprise and/or preautomated records		√
Workflow management for optically stored documents		√
Long-term storage of patient care documents	√	√
Electronic signature	√	√
Fax		√
Electronic mail		√
Input of clinician notes	√	√
Provides direct clinician use for patient care	√	√
Provides access to longitudinal patient records across sites	√	√

© First Consulting Group 1998

Computerized Patient Records

Today, a healthcare organization that has automated over 20 percent of the inpatient and outpatient record has surpassed its competitors. Most organizations have automated only 10 to 20 percent of the record, usually the face sheet, lab results, and some transcription. One prestigious organization leapt ahead by automating nearly 80 percent of some inpatient records; yet the same organization continues to maintain significant paper-based records, especially in the outpatient areas, as shown in Table 13.2.

Clearly, without imaging technology, healthcare organizations will continue to swim in paper for the foreseeable future, and access to patient information will remain dependent upon paper-based records.

TABLE 13.2. Percentage of automated records for one organization.

Discipline/service	% Automated	% Paper
Chemotherapy	81%	19%
Esophagitis	62%	38%
Coronary heart failure	66%	34%
Embolic stroke	63%	37%
Pneumonia	79%	21%
Hypokalemia	68%	32%
Behavioral health —Depression with	37%	63%
GYN-TAH	54%	46%
Vaginal delivery	49%	51%
Newborns	47%	53%

© First Consulting Group 1998

Workflow

What is workflow? According to Marshak (1995), it is "applying technology to business processes—in other words, using computers to help groups of people get their work done" (p. 225). Workflow software addresses the series of tasks required for processing documents throughout the organization, ultimately making information available on the user's desktop. It does so based on the organization's rules, procedures, and business objectives. This is, in essence, facilitating business processes—and the key to operational improvements and cost savings. Clearly, workflow technology is the component of document management that offers health care the greatest potential benefits.

How does it work? Let's look to banking, one of the first industries to make major use of workflow technology in process redesign. According to several studies, some banks took two weeks to process each credit card application, while the actual tasks involved required less than 30 minutes.

Sadly, most healthcare executives can cite examples of similar processes in health care, with its many manual and paper-based processes. Healthcare organizations thus stand to benefit significantly from workflow development and utilization across the enterprise. Once processes like billing and registration are redesigned, document management (primarily the workflow component) can enhance them to eliminate the manual inefficiencies accumulated over the years.

Consider one organization suffering nearly $500,000 per year in lost Medicaid reimbursement due to missing and misplaced ambulance forms. Planned changes in workflow call for automatically routing scanned ambulance forms to the business office based on patient type (i.e., Medicaid) located in the hospital information system's ADT interface and the indexing of form type (i.e., ambulance form).

We believe the real benefits come when workflow is applied enterprise-wide to reengineered processes, including those beyond the realm of the computerized patient record.

- **Business office.** Currently many business offices use imaging to capture the portion of the billing record that is not automated, such as consents. Few use workflow technology to route information and documents, such as bills and explanations of benefits (EOBs), to the appropriate clerk based on the organization's rules. For example, all Aetna bills with an alpha split of A-P can be electronically routed to clerk A except for bills for employees with Aetna coverage, which are routed to the manager.

- **Human resources.** Imaging can help store and integrate employee records not resident on the human resources information system. Many organizations maintain multiple nonintegrated employee records within human resources, employee health, medical staff office, nurse staffing, and individual departments for licensure and accreditation. Workflow can help track resumes and maintain comments offered about a candidate in the event the candidate reapplies. It can automatically transmit lab and other test results, such as mandatory tuberculosis tests, directly to the employee's "folder," eliminating the need to route paper.

- **Risk management.** Updating departmental policies and procedures is an ongoing process. When an updated policy is distributed, the organization has to maintain the replaced policy in the event a claim is made against the time the replaced policy was in effect. It is not unusual for departments to "misplace" the replaced policy, potentially placing the organization at risk during any claim or potential lawsuit. Document management can store all current and previous editions of policies and procedures so they will be available to all personnel at any image-enabled workstation.
- **Home health.** Despite efforts to automate, home health continues to be intensely paper-based. Imaging offers immediate benefits. If physician offices are linked to the document management system, records can be accessed electronically, eliminating the need to copy and mail all information generated about the patient over the past 60 days. Workflow can provide electronic alerts and reminders based on the organization's "rules." For example, agencies track driver's license renewals and maintain updated copies of car insurance policies for employees who commute to visit patients. Workflow software can automate this process, which is typically manual, and send electronic alerts regarding employees with expiring licenses or insurance.

Other areas like materials management, accounts payable, and clinics could use document management to enhance operations. Organizations considering the applicability of the technology should think about its potential benefits in every area of the enterprise.

Capabilities of Document Management

The healthcare industry has yet to understand the intricacies of document management. To derive maximum value, we need to go beyond the file and retrieve activities inherent in imaging. The application of workflow technology can help organizations to remain key players in the marketplace. Robust workflow can provide operational efficiencies and reduce costs; it can also improve access to patient management and clinical information across the continuum of care, enhancing patient service.

Adding Value

We believe that adding value through technology requires a strong understanding of business and clinical processes. Applying technology to a poor manual process results in an inefficient automated process with no significant return on investment. Whether implementing a call center or document management or any other emerging or established technology, always evaluate and, if necessary, redesign processes before automating them.

References

Le Doeuf, M. 1987. *How to Win Customers and Keep Them for Life*. West Lafayette, Ind.: Purdue University.

Marshak, R. 1995. "Perspectives on Workflow." In *The Workflow Paradigm*. 2d ed. Ed. L. Fisher. Lighthouse Point, Fla.: Future Strategies.

14

Implications and Direction

JAMES REEP AND PHILIP LOHMAN

In the sometimes-harsh climate of competitive markets, healthcare organizations have focused on taking practical measures to ensure their future. As in any attempt to anticipate the direction of change, some measures have proved more effective than others, but the attempts have all been necessary and have contributed to the healthcare industry's foundation of shared knowledge and skills. The purpose of this chapter is to set forth considerations for strategic management in health care as we enter the next century and to suggest specific initiatives and techniques that we believe hold promise.

The Permanence of Change in Health Care

Despite the hopes of some executives and physicians, there will be no return to the "good old days" in health care. In the U.S. and other advanced economies, the healthcare industry is now driven by forces that it does not control, from politics and economics to the environment and medicine itself. (For a full discussion of these forces, see Chapter 2.) A single field of advance, such as our newfound knowledge of the human genetic code, promises to have unforeseeable—but unquestionably seismic—effects on how we predict, diagnose, and treat hereditary diseases and diseases that have a component of genetic predisposition.

The consequence of this dynamism is an increasingly Protean healthcare industry. A few years ago, we could tick off the major sectors of the industry—doctors, hospitals, health plans and other insurers—on a few fingers. Today we confront a bewildering blur of business models and organizational types, proving once again that evolution leads to specialization. Another, more momentous consequence is change so fast-paced that it is outstripping the established ways of dealing with it. Markets are transformed faster than we can build the enterprises to serve them. Joseph Schumpeter's "creative destruction," wreaked by the competitive market, is leaving the landscape littered with business strategies that were obsolete before they could be implemented.

From Institution to Process

Adapting to the onrush of change in the healthcare market will require a true paradigm shift—a change not in how we *do* things, but in how we *understand* them (Kuhn 1962). Traditionally, health care has been understood as a function of stable or slowly evolving institutions—the hospital, the independent medical practice, the research institute, the insurance company, the family. Healthcare strategies were designed to maximize the efficiency of these institutions, the permanence of which was never questioned.

Today, however, the economic circumstances of these institutions are changing, and information technology is dissolving the barriers between organizations everywhere. Increasingly, health care is being designed with an eye to the goals to be achieved—a change that became inevitable once quality was redefined in terms of outcomes—with each function within the overall process being performed by whoever does it most cost-effectively. For example, the integration of care delivery has led restructuring integrated delivery organizations to outsource not only administrative and support functions, but also components of care—in some cases, to their own competitors.

Building for Impermanence

The net result of these changes is that the "bricks and mortar" investments of yesterday are becoming the process investments of today. The intense focus on clinical outcomes and service satisfaction as competitive advantages, combined with the ongoing pressure to hold down costs, has yielded a simple rule: any expenditure that does not add value at the level of core clinical and business processes is increasingly suspect.

While this concentration on value appears to have promise for making the U.S healthcare delivery system much more cost efficient, it has had a number of less desirable side effects, notably the frequently high level of stress felt almost everywhere in health care as departments are dissolved, job descriptions are changed, and relationships once thought permanent are placed in seemingly perpetual renegotiation.

Agenda for Healthcare Leadership

If healthcare executives are to succeed in such an environment, we believe they must radically rethink their own objectives and roles. Specifically, they must concentrate on a small number of basic issues: finding the sources of value to the market, serving new markets, serving old markets better, identifying and serving stakeholders, and adapting to the emergence of the consumer as a major force in health care.

Finding Sources of Value to the Market

Competitive markets are ruthless in their ability to winnow out competitors that do not provide superior value. The difficulty is knowing, in the turbulent healthcare environment, what the sources of the healthcare organization's value are. These may be less visible than we think. We tend to see markets in terms of individual, insurer-reimbursed services (for example, cardiovascular services in a market that lacks them) and specific populations (such as Medicare). Yet it is likely that value will soon be measured less by what health care is delivered and to whom. As consumers gain a greater say in the operation of healthcare markets, the real measure of value will be *how* health care is delivered.

While it has been a long time coming, the "consumer revolution" in health care is on the verge of reality. Employers are realizing they can manage healthcare costs with less administrative overhead by separating administration from financing and letting employees make their own informed decisions about care. In Minneapolis, for example, the Buyers Healthcare Action Group rates providers on understandable scales of cost and quality, and this information is made directly available to employees of participating employers. Although the employers offer a variety of incentives to choose high-quality, low-cost providers, employees are otherwise free to choose any provider. Financial services companies such as State Street Boston Corporation and consultants such as Watson Wyatt Worldwide are teaming to offer complete administrative and reimbursement services to employers who wish to outsource employee healthcare: the employee will get an annual check or voucher for care, will receive advice on care plans and providers, and will be free to make the best deal he or she can.

These signs are early but portentous, since these initiatives offer both employers and employees an almost irresistible proposition. Employers get predictable premium outlays for health care and sharply lowered administrative burdens. Employees, no longer tied to employer decisions about health plans and newly empowered as consumers, can voice their wants forcefully: an unhappy experience will result not in an appeal to a health plan or an angry letter to a benefits manager or union representative, but in the departure of a customer. Conversely, healthcare enterprises that treat consumers with care, in terms of both clinical and nonclinical services, will have a decisive competitive advantage.

This means that health plans that have spent years learning one market—employers—will now find themselves facing an entirely new one—consumers. Care providers whose deficiencies cost their plans members will quickly find themselves without contracts. Value will be redefined by consumer demands, and healthcare enterprises will survive only by meeting them.

To meet consumer demands, healthcare organizations will have to develop capabilities that have long been routine in other industries but are still new to health care: consumer market analysis, customer communications, customer education, customer service, and brand management. Healthcare organizations will have to be able to explain differences in plan costs and benefits in the customer's language, provide quality information in ways that customers can understand, offer access at the customer's convenience, and resolve problems quickly and courteously. None of this will be easy; all of it will be necessary. Those organizations—like Intermountain Health Care in Salt Lake City, which bases its process redesign work around a single concept: the "quality of the patient experience"—will have a head start.

In this environment, healthcare organizations may find that their value to the consumer resides in unexpected places—for example, the ability to:

- integrate lifestyle/wellness programs or alternative medicine with traditional medicine
- offer customers convenient access to care at work
- excel in customer health education
- empower customers with information technology and custom-designed, self-managed programs for chronic conditions.

Managing the Transition to New Markets

The transition to the consumer-driven healthcare market of the next decade will be complex, but it need not be difficult. Healthcare organizations that have aggressively moved toward quality reporting, such as Kaiser Health Plan and the provider members of Cleveland Health Quality Choice, will have an advantage; so will those that have undertaken fundamental restructuring to better serve their existing customers, as has Rocky Mountain Administrative Services Corporation, the parent company of Colorado Blue Cross–Blue Shield. Organizations that have experimented with innovative care delivery models—provider-sponsored networks, for example—will benefit from their experience (good or bad), as will those, like Group Health of Puget Sound, who have begun to develop custom healthcare insurance products for the consumer market (Corkrum 1998).

Innovation, however, must be built on a solid foundation of basics: clinical and administrative integration, implementation of clinical and business best practices, cost structures that permit competitive pricing, rigorous monitoring of clinical and service quality. Healthcare organizations must shed what industry critic Jeff Goldsmith has called "industrial thinking"—the belief that assembling massive organizations and pursuing controlling market share will yield satisfactory returns. Rather, they need to develop a flexible contracting strategy, invest in their core competencies and successful enterprises, and shed enterprises where they clearly cannot create value. Goldsmith's conclusion anticipates the emerging consumer market:

> The most important integration that needs to occur is integration people notice when they use the product or services. . .that it saves them money, or that they get services twice as fast, or that their needs are met in a way that they can measure in their own lives. (Goldsmith 1997, p. 8)

In many cases, then, healthcare enterprises will help build a foundation for serving their new markets by undertaking the changes that allow them to serve their current markets better.

Identifying and Serving Stakeholders

There is a growing awareness in the United States that business enterprises (defined broadly to include not-for-profits) have, in addition to stockholders, communities of "stakeholders"—i.e., people who have an interest in the actions of the enterprise. Such academics as Edward Freeman (1984) and Thomas Donaldson and Lee E. Preston (1995) have spurred lively debate about the nature and extent of the enterprise's obligations to stakeholders. However, it is fairly clear that in many industries, considering stakeholder interests is prudent whether this move is obligatory or not. This is particularly true in health care, which is highly susceptible to organized political pressure and community disaffection.

The community of stakeholders in health care is quite large and includes health plan members, patients, employees, and members of local communities. Of these groups, the one whose interests are least likely to be addressed in existing organizational strategy is the last—local community members.

Members of local communities typically have a wide range of interests in the organization's behavior: traffic around large facilities, for example, or concern about handling of biohazardous waste. In each of these areas of concern, the organization has both short-term and long-term interests, and will need to gather and process the information to distinguish between the two and to implement its response.

The most common interest, however, is likely to be in community wellness, an area where the community's interests and the organization's, regarded in the long term, are likely to coincide. Promoting community wellness through free education programs, outreach, and screening (e.g., diabetes, mammograms, hypertension) will inevitably lead to additional costs for both the programs and for uncompensated care. However, it is precisely the sort of community benefit that healthcare organizations are best qualified to provide and, over the long term, to share.

There are several keys to successful community wellness promotion. First, programs should not be "add-ons" for Saturday afternoons; they should be part of the overall strategy of the organization. Second, they should be planned and designed with the same concern for information management and efficient process design as the organization's other activities. Above all, the healthcare organization must make concern for stakeholder interests—regardless of how it responds in any particular case—a standard component of organizational strategy.

Doubtless, there are many other influences that will touch health care in the coming decade—medical, demographical, political, and so on (we can, for example, anticipate a growing trend toward national standards of care for managed care), but few will so directly alter the structure of the industry as the growing influence of consumers and stakeholders—consumers through the marketplace, and stakeholders through the community, the legislatures, and the courts.

The Tools of Healthcare Leadership

To adapt to these changes, there are certain directions in which healthcare leadership will need to develop in the coming decades. These follow hard upon the changes that leadership in this industry has already made—broadly, from a social service/institutional caretaker role to that of entrepreneur and business strategist. These new roles will be further modified as health care evolves and as the fund of executive knowledge grows.

The Chief Executive Officer as Team Leader

While there is a perpetual debate over leadership styles and characteristics (charismatic/transformational, task-oriented/relationship-oriented, etc.), there is less debate over the situation that confronts healthcare leaders: a turbulent industry with great complexity and discontinuity, and with a staggering amount of information to be processed and applied. There is also a younger, multicultural generation of management that has matured in a very different world from that of its elders. Younger managers and executives are, in general, entrepreneurial, informal, technology-oriented, and accustomed to having a good deal of latitude, for which they are prepared to be accountable. They do not function well in bureaucratic or authoritarian environments. Consequently, the leadership style of a generation ago is usually off the mark in today's environment.

Recent research has shown that, rather than act from inborn traits of personality (e.g., "charismatic"), successful business leaders "adopt the approach that will best meet the needs of the organization and the business situation at hand" (Farkas and Wetlaufer 1996, p. 111). In health care, as in many other industries, the "situation at hand" is adaptation to a radically different set of market forces and stakeholder expectations. This requires leaders to break a habit that got most of them where they are—providing solutions—and to learn a new set of behaviors that create and sustain an environment in which individuals can undertake the work of adapting the organization to the conditions it now faces (Heifetz and Laurie 1997). The resulting style is more supportive and coordinating than controlling, and places a heavy emphasis on clearly defining the adaptive challenge, fine-tuning motivational stress while empowering employees, promoting and protecting diverse views, and providing support—and, where necessary, cover—to change agents and internal critics.

This leadership style is particularly apposite to health care, with its polymorphous organizations and its sometimes-fractious mix of medical, technical, managerial, and entrepreneurial cultures. It is also essential for the development of the diverse, specialty-based teams that are becoming the key to effective management in rapidly changing industries.

This style is in sharp contrast to the benevolent autocrats of a generation ago, and, although hard data are scarce, many healthcare industry participants are beginning to see the emergence, on the job, of this new echelon of leaders.

The Pivotal Role of Organizational and Professional Culture

Traditionally, there has been exactly one cultural issue in health care: understanding, working with, and occasionally manipulating physicians. In this context, the "physician culture" was (and in many quarters, still is) seen as an obstacle to the achievement of larger goals, a promoter of narrowness and an intransigent guild mentality. Certainly, the tension between physicians and others was often real and material (regarding issues of compensation, for example), but often it was illusory and a waste of energy. It usually stemmed from a fundamental misunderstanding of the role that culture plays, not only among physicians, but in other groups of healthcare workers, technicians, and professionals.

Indeed, the rule that evolution leads to complexity and specialization applies to cultures just as it does to plants and animals. As healthcare organizations have evolved and grown more complex, they have fostered a growing number of cultures—broadly defined as shared (but usually implicit) beliefs and attitudes about meaning and value.

In leading the healthcare organization, it is important to remember several things about culture. First, cultures are in large measure a structure of *meaning* through which we understand events, language, and actions. (A simple example: to a nurse, "participation" in a clinical decision means having input; to a doctor, it means having a veto.) Consequently, addressing people by circumventing their culture is less effective than translating communications into their terms.

Second, each of us participates in multiple cultures within an organization. In a for-profit physician hospital organization, for example, a physician may, as a member of the organization, be part of a "customer culture," but as a physician, he or she is a member of a professional culture. These overlaps create additional complexity, but they also present additional opportunities for understanding and cooperation.

If professional cultures are understood and addressed thoughtfully, their existence will offer healthcare leadership an important key. Since cultures present long-term structures of understanding and value, they can be effective means of communicating, organizing, and managing. Understanding what a group values allows organizational leaders to position goals and create incentives—often in terms of the sources of identity and emotional support that the culture provides for its members. Physicians, for example, have a profound emotional investment in their hard-won identity as healers. Information and telecommunication specialists are more than just "techies" with an odd vocabulary; their culture bears a robust "can-do" spirit and a deep esprit de corps. The successful leader in health care knows that the way to understand and motivate these groups—and others, such as clinical technologists and nurses—is to speak their own language (Gross and Lohman 1997).

In some cases, cultures can pose obstacles to accomplishing specific goals; this most often occurs when a decision is seen as a judgment on the relative importance of group interests rather than on the facts. In these cases, it is important to ensure that decisions are data-driven and made in the interests of the organization as a whole. Applying this principle serves not only to establish a shared and objective basis of understanding, but also to synthesize different viewpoints.

Building the Executive Team

While leadership may not depend on inherent traits of personality, it is nevertheless a specialized skill that demands viewing a large, complex healthcare organization from a certain point of view, which we usually refer to as "strategic."

This point of view addresses the broad characteristics of the organization's environment—its market(s), its strengths and weaknesses, its legal and political situation, its personality and culture. It is by definition different from the "operational" point of view, which attends to the effectiveness and efficiency of specific processes and activities within the organization in meeting the goals set by strategy. Nevertheless, a solid understanding of operations and a "grip" on core processes must be accessible *to* the leader, even if they are not a characteristic *of* the leader.

In the past, this link has typically been provided by a "first mate," a senior executive who understands both strategy and operations and can link the two effectively. This practice is changing as CEOs find that they need a link to operations that is broader, and input to strategy that is more diverse, than that provided by a single executive. This is consistent with the general trend of management away from hierarchy and authority-based leadership and toward leadership that is looser and more competence- and situation-based.

Some critics argue that top management teams, as successors to the traditional hierarchically organized leadership group, have become something of a fad. Many so-called teams, the argument goes, are not really teams at all, simply modishly renamed hierarchical groups. Real teams require unity of purpose, a lot of time, and mutual accountability. They have shifting leadership, depending on the task at hand. Coordination consumes time and makes teams less efficient than traditional structures (Katzenbach 1997).

There are, however, strong arguments for the team approach in health care, either alone or as an alternative mode for special circumstances. The industry's agenda has many components—restructuring around core processes, integrating administrative, financial, and clinical information into coherent process guidance and performance reporting, learning and dealing with new markets, and bringing multiple professional and technical cultures into alignment. All of these components demand an intensely interactive process among a diverse set of top leaders and, to a considerable degree, the relaxation of hierarchy within the organization. Above all, they demand the ability to deliberate fully but execute swiftly once a consensus is reached.

In the long run, most successful healthcare organizations will probably wind up redefining both teamwork and leadership at the top. The most successful CEOs will be those who are skilled at developing and articulating a strategic vision and goals, developing and coordinating subordinates, and leading quickly to consensus. In the most successful teams, members will be able to move in and out of situational leadership roles as circumstances demand: the chief medical officer leads today, the chief financial officer tomorrow.

The Next Generation of Leaders

As the healthcare industry passes through its current stage of evolution and into the next, the development of tomorrow's leaders becomes ever more critical. The industry, we should recall, has recently suffered from a serious deficiency of suitable leadership as it moved from fee-for-service into managed care. Many organizations were unprepared at the executive level for the wrenching effects of this change in the market, despite the fact that the signs had begun appearing in the early 1970s and the compelling logic of managed care was clearly visible.

Today, while we cannot answer some of the questions that loom in the industry's future (how, for example, *will* the federal government fund Medicare in the long term?), we do know a lot about what will be required to meet them. Healthcare organizations, by entering the competitive marketplace, have committed themselves to consumer sovereignty, with all that implies: market discipline, change, and permanent restructuring. Consequently, the next generation of leaders will need both the standard leadership skills (goal orientation, ability to prioritize, and so on) and the ability to tolerate radical discontinuities and find the keys to action in immense quantities of information. Above all, new leaders will need to grasp in an instinctive way how organizations must adapt to markets.

The implications of this profile for new leaders in health care suggest that the traditional paths of leadership development will change. Historically, healthcare leaders have been developed within an organizational context and with a strong emphasis on institutional loyalty and commitment (many still are, particularly in the Roman Catholic healthcare tradition). In this context, the organization would make a conscious effort to provide mentoring from established senior executives.

Today, however, both circumstances and people have changed. The arrival of the global economy, with its radical disruption of traditional economic relationships, has reduced employment security throughout the economy at precisely the moment that the baby boomers, notorious for their skepticism, are arriving at positions of leadership. Moreover, there is the special problem of health care, where industry turbulence has disrupted many careers and severed institutional loyalties wholesale.

The next generation of leaders, consequently, is likely to emerge from different sources, develop in different ways, and lead differently than the last generation. The growth of "free agency" indicates that careers are now largely in the hands of their "owners" and that those who aspire to leadership should expect to be on their own in preparing for it. Consequently, leadership development is likely to be less a matter of cultivating talent than of recognizing it and opening the door for its exercise and shaping it toward the organization's goals at the moment.

The Uses and Nonuses of Information Technology

The experience of the healthcare industry with information technology (IT) has been, in many respects, a difficult one. In the mid-1980s, beginning from a level of automation well below that of other industries, health care turned to information technology in an attempt to accomplish a number of things simultaneously. Information technology was applied to integrating organizations by linking departments, reducing manual labor costs in clerical areas, tracking utilization, and similar routine activities. In most cases, the results were less than desired. The technology of the time wasn't up to the demands, much effort was expended on marginal goals, and inadequate attention was paid to integrating and rationalizing overall processes. Despite some successes, a growing cloud of peer skepticism gathered over IT departments. In retrospect, little was accomplished by information technology because relatively little was demanded of it.

Fortunately, the demands of managed care, like the prospect of being hanged, in Samuel Johnson's famous anecdote, have tended to concentrate the health-care industry's mind wonderfully. The need for radical cost reduction and the requirements of serving entirely new markets have forced a wholesale rethinking of the role of information and telecommunications technology in health care.

Clearly, using information technology in isolation to automate individual steps in a multistep process accomplishes little more than adding automated costs to manual costs and little or nothing to overall process or enterprise performance. Information technology is most effective when it is used as a solvent to dissolve established, dysfunctional structures and as a catalyst for end-to-end process redesign. The implications of this for the technology and the organizations that use it are profound: *information technology succeeds to the extent that it is flexible, intuitive to use, and able to empower people*. Organizations—especially in health care—succeed with technology to the extent that they employ it as the basic medium of operational leverage and control.

Opportunities and Pitfalls in Process Improvement

In the last two decades, innovations in strategy and management have seemed to follow a standard sequence. First, they are announced in management books or academic journals, whereupon they generate a wave of favorable comment. Second, they are hailed by popularizers and the business press as "revolutionary breakthroughs" that will work near-miracles. Third, they are implemented carefully at a few organizations, where they meet with moderate success, and hastily at many more, where they inevitably fail. Finally, the press denounces the innovation as "another management fad" and the whole thing is forgotten. What is unfortunate about this chain of events, of course, is that the innovation never really has a chance to succeed.

One of these innovations is reengineering. Originally associated with the work of Michael Hammer (Hammer 1996; Hammer and Champy 1993) and, in health care, with J. Philip Lathrop (1993), reengineering has been pilloried by a number of failures and by growing skepticism and confusion. Much of the skepticism stems from doubts that the radical change proposed by reengineering is really necessary and the belief that incremental change (the Japanese *kaizen*) is safer and more controllable.

Clearly, there is no hard rule for this decision, since the prescription depends on the diagnosis delivered by the market. Some situations (e.g., a pooling-of-assets merger or a "near-death experience" in the market) clearly suggest that reengineering will be required, while others (e.g., poor performance of one strategic business unit) suggest that a more moderate approach is prudent. It is essential, however, to recognize that most legacy organizations of the fee-for-service era are poorly adapted for managed care, and that, as the pace of market change accelerates, many of these organizations will find that radical change will be the price of survival.

A more pervasive doubt about reengineering is the manageability of the entire process. Certainly, there are risks involved in reengineering, as there are with any human enterprise. However, these have to be balanced against the risks of doing either nothing or too little. As a practical matter, risk is an inverse function of good management. Following experience-based "best practices" can dramatically improve the odds: clarity on the business case and degree of change it dictates; adoption of a specific, proven methodology; full commitment and active involvement of top leadership; recognition of the size of the capital investment required; integrated use of information and telecommunications technology as the catalyst for designing core processes and empowering staff; tracking of progress and results with integrated clinical and business performance measures; and willingness to move quickly once the analysis is done. As in everything else, planning is the easy part; successful organizations focus their efforts on execution.

Reengineering is not a panacea—it will not, for example, save a bad business strategy—but it is a great deal more than a fad. With proper management, it can deliver solid results.

Surviving Success, Benefiting from Failure

Turbulent markets raise the stakes for any strategy: the potential for both gains and losses increases. This tends to reward entrepreneurial aggressiveness and punish timidity, since enterprises that move quickly to adapt will usually fare better than those that remain on the sidelines waiting for the situation to become clearer. This does not mean that an organization should plunge blindly ahead. It *does* mean that while aggressiveness may not guarantee superior performance, timidity almost certainly ensures relatively poor performance.

Unfortunately, aggressiveness comes with its own risks since new ventures often fail, presenting the enterprise with a classic problem: how to deal with failure. The key is that failure is always an opportunity in itself—to learn more about the market and the organization. Success, on the other hand, creates the more subtle danger of simply doing more of the same on the implicit assumption that the market will remain as it is. Oddly enough, organizations may find they must learn to survive success more than failure.

An instructive example of these principles is the experience of group practices with capitation. While many of the early experiments with capitated contracts resulted in financial losses for the providers, the groups that pursued these aggressively were able to learn to manage utilization and other costs in a relatively forgiving environment and bring their practices back into the black with succeeding contracts. Groups that resisted taking capitated contracts until they were compelled to by circumstances had a much steeper learning curve to climb—and at a time when capitation rates, in many cases, were lower.

Failure, ironically, may become a virtue. In *The Organization of the Future*, Deepak Sethi points out that "the organization of the future will *demand* mistakes and failures, as proof that its people are committed to risk taking and innovation" (Sethi 1997, p. 233) For health care, an inherently conservative industry, this will be a momentous change.

Vision as a Tactical Tool

Despite its general acceptance as a strategic tool, "visioning" in health care, as in other industries, has been a frequent target of good-humored mockery. This is largely because of its vaguely religious overtones—the image of the "CEO receiving a vision" in a sort of trance is irresistible to cartoonists and commentators. However, if taken seriously as criticism, this viewpoint on visioning has some merit. Strategic visions are implicitly treated as a kind of Platonic idea, visible to the highly evolved and communicated to the rest through a managerial priesthood in the form of performance goals. Though these goals theoretically support core values, they are constantly in danger of becoming lip service—or worse, at the desk level, just another management fad. As Tom Peters observed in *Liberation Management,* "all good ideas eventually get oversold" (Peters 1997, pp. 616–617).

On the contrary, the organization's vision is a valuable if not crucial tool in the emerging healthcare market. As a means of strategic thinking, it allows the creation of a concrete—if imaginary—future in the form of a coherent set of goals and states the values on which the organization rests. Visioning, however, has been largely neglected as a *tactical* tool because too many organizations lose the connection between the vision and the daily activities that get the organization's work done. This explains the cynicism that sometimes greets visioning at the departmental level.

As healthcare organizations become less monolithic and more networked, and employees are empowered and expected to find solutions through teams rather than through channels, the organization's vision must take on some of the directive role traditionally played by managers and supervisors. The employee who understands the vision, shares the values, *and believes on good evidence that the organization takes both of them seriously* will be far more likely to make an effective contribution than one who does not. *The challenge is for the organization to live up to them by making tactical decisions that explicitly support them.*

The healthcare industry, with its history of service and its ethic of compassion, has always attracted those who are motivated by transcendent ideals. This has been one of the more difficult passages for the industry as it makes the transition to competitive markets.

Managing Risk and Cost in Information Technology

In the healthcare industry, part of the legacy of information technology's early stumbles has been the abiding perception that IT projects pose an inordinate level of risk. This perception has not been dissipated by the growing reliance of the healthcare industry on automated solutions. Certainly, the application of information and telecommunications technology carries some degree of risk—as does any human enterprise—but we have also learned a great deal about how to manage and control projects to minimize it.

If we define risk as the likelihood that the technology project will fail to achieve its goals, it becomes clearer that there are levels of risk. The first is pure technology risk, i.e., that the technology simply won't work—the software will be full of bugs, the hardware will fail, and the network won't carry the level of traffic claimed for it. The second level of risk has to do with the project itself. Even if the technology works, it is possible that the project will fail as a technical effort—the conversion will never take place or will fail, the application will not be as useful to users as originally thought. The third level of risk is *operational.* The operational goals for which the project was conceived may not be reached, medication errors may not go down, patient waiting times may increase, supply inventory costs may go up.

It is evident that the last two levels of risk are not, strictly speaking, technological. Rather, they are risks associated with *management.* In fact, contemporary information and telecommunications technology is highly reliable and increasingly adaptive to a wide range of requirements. What is too often missing is a clear conception of the project, a definition of operational gains to be achieved, and the skills—some of them highly specialized—to manage the work.

In other words, the IT project as traditionally defined—i.e., implementing packaged solutions to "automate" a single manual process like patient registration—is almost completely obsolete. Such projects, no matter how many there are, rarely achieve significant overall operational gains. Success *in terms of organizational goals* is more likely if the project is conceived as an *operational effectiveness* project, with a clear definition of overall process change and operational goals to be achieved through the appropriate mix of reengineering and information/telecommunications technology.

With the project thus redefined, there are a number of steps that the organization can take to manage risk associated with the technology being employed. First, it can ensure that it has made an explicit decision on the level of risk to be accepted and that this has been measured against the anticipated benefits of the project (well-established technologies are typically less powerful but also generally less risky). Second, it can ensure that it has the right set of skills to support the technology it intends to implement; these must either be acquired by hiring or developed by retraining. Third, it can require the vendor to share project risk by writing the contract so that payments to the vendor are linked to specific milestones, rather than being paid monthly, and that incentives are provided for specific performance items (however, the organizations should be cautious about signing "codevelopment" or "beta site" contracts). Finally, it can pilot new technologies—one large clinic in the Midwest has created a "usability lab" for this purpose.

The risk of new technologies is real but probably overstated; the risks of misapplication or failure to realize value are a good deal more pressing.

Realizing Value in Information Technology

Realizing a return on information technology has been both a hotly debated issue and a major practical problem, especially in health care. For more than two decades, healthcare organizations have made investments in information technology which, while small by comparison with other industries, often did not provide even the modest benefit consistent with the investment. Projects undertaken with ambitious intentions and high hopes failed to meet their goals, were superseded by other projects, or were simply abandoned. The anticipated impacts on cost and operational performance were less than expected or none at all.

There are many explanations for this, but here are some of the principal causes: paying insufficient attention to organizational structure, work flows, and people; failing to use information technology to address end-to-end process issues; purchasing technology that took so long to implement that the business case for its use changed before the system was operational; spending too much on applications and not enough on network infrastructure; not defining operational goals or not enforcing progress toward them; trying to (in Peter Drucker's words) "feed problems" by automating processes that already delivered poor results; and concentrating on low-return financial processes (e.g., billing, payroll, general ledger) rather than high-return clinical processes.

This list suggests the basic strategies for maximizing return:

- Define operational goals first, then design the processes to meet them, applying technology as necessary to make the processes work as designed.
- Concentrate on high-leverage areas, such as clinical processes that can be redesigned to lower costs of care.
- Concentrate first on processes that bring in revenue from external customers.
- Develop management control systems that link financial and clinical information.
- Buy technology with a high degree of inbuilt flexibility.
- Build the network infrastructure before it is needed, not after.
- Concentrate technology investments on breakthrough targets, not incremental improvements.
- Manage information across the organization, not department by department.
- Above all, remember that systems do not create value—*people do.*

Tactics for improving the performance of information and telecommunications technology include the following: establishing uniform data definitions and standards; using business performance metrics rather than technical metrics as a measure of technology performance; estimating the cost of IT projects by full life cycle rather than by initial capital outlay; and outsourcing selectively without being "kidnapped" by an outsource. Throughout the project's duration, keep operations managers and executives (including physicians) accountable for project success. (For a highly detailed treatment of the topic of technology value realization, see Strassman 1997.)

Information technology represents a rapidly growing percentage of healthcare organizations' operating budgets. If properly managed, it can pay off in solid improvements in basic processes and operating performance.

Management, Management, Management

A common saying is that problems are simply opportunities in disguise. If this saying is true anywhere, it is in health care. The disappearance of the healthcare industry's stability and the near-chaotic restructuring it is undergoing have forced a number of essential changes almost simultaneously. We are assembling a growing body of knowledge on what works and what doesn't in managed care. We are defining a growing repertoire of business strategies. We are sharing the advances in management developed in other industries and are developing many of our own. We have powerful information technologies available, and more are arriving in a virtual avalanche of innovation. We are perfecting the tools of process improvement. What remains for us as an industry is to develop a way to make all of these components work together smoothly.

While every project is unique, there are some general principles for integrating the many components of a major reengineering project. The overriding principle is this: *the root of all performance improvement is the will to manage for it.* This dictates common, objective, measurable results—improved services, reduced cycle times, reduced time-to-market, improved quality of care, and lower costs. It also dictates a closed cycle of plan, act, evaluate, replan, with attention to some specific tactical considerations:

- Leadership must *lead.* The CEO and, if necessary, chairperson of the board must be actively involved, not merely supply "visibility."
- The project takes precedence over everything else, period.
- It is essential that all involved parties understand the role, capabilities, and limitations of information technology; however, they must *not* let the project direction be set by the information systems department. Information technology must remain an enabler, not an independent variable.
- Reengineering must be driven by the market and the organization's mission in the market, not by internal imperatives or politics.
- Empowerment *means* empowerment. The organization cannot half-trust its employees. Define goals and accountability clearly, give employees the resources, and turn them loose.

• Above all, remember this: health care is the most humane of all industries; its whole reason for being is caring. While we cannot eliminate the stress and pain of change, we must do whatever we can to help others deal with it.

References

Corkrum, D.S. 1998. "Mass Customization at Group Health Co-op," *Healthcare Strategist*, January, pp. 6–8.

Donaldson, T. and L.E. Preston. 1995. "The Stakeholder Theory of the Corporation—Concepts, Evidence and Implications," *Academy of Management Review* 20(1), pp. 65–91.

Farkas, C.M. and S. Wetlaufer. 1996. "The Ways Chief Executive Officers Lead," *Harvard Business Review*, May–June, pp. 110–125.

Freeman, E. 1984. *Strategic Management, A Stakeholder Approach*. Marshfield, Mass., Pitman.

Goldsmith, J. 1997. "IDS Survival Strategies," *Medical Network Strategy Report*, July, pp. 3–8.

Gross, M. and P. Lohman. 1997. "The Technology and Tactics of Physician Integration," *Journal of the Healthcare Information and Management Systems Society* 11(2), Summer, pp. 26--32.

Hammer, M. 1996. *Beyond Reengineering*. New York: HarperBusiness.

Hammer, M. and J. Champy. 1993. *Reengineering the Corporation*. New York: HarperBusiness.

Heifetz, R. and D.L. Laurei. 1997. "The Work of Leadership," *Harvard Business Review*, January-February, pp. 124–135.

Katzenbach J.R. 1997. "The Myth of the Top Management Team," *Harvard Business Review*, November–December, pp. 82–91.

Kuhn, T. 1970. *The Structure of Scientific Revolutions*. Chicago: University of Chicago Press.

Lathrop, J. Philip. 1993. *Restructuring Health Care*. San Francisco: Jossey-Bass.

Peters, T. 1992. *Liberation Management—Necessary Disorganization for the Nanosecond Nineties*. New York: Fawcett Columbine.

Sethi, D. 1997. "The Seven R's of Self Esteem." In *The Organization of the Future,* ed. M. Goldsmith. San Francisco: Jossey-Bass.

Shapiro, E. 1995. "Reengineering and the Labors of Hercules," *Fad Surfing in the Boardroom*. Reading, Mass.: Addison-Wesley, pp. 183–195.

Strassman, P.A. 1997. *The Squandered Computer: Evaluating the Business Alignment of Information Technologies*. New Canaan, Conn.: Information Economics Press.

Index

Contributors

Robert K. Antczak
Technical Master, First Consulting Group, Coventry, RI, USA

Marion J. Ball, EdD
Vice President, First Consulting Group, Baltimore, MD, USA
<mball@fcgnet.com>

David Beaulieu
Vice President, First Consulting Group, Waltham, MA, USA
<dbeaulieu@fcgnet.com>

Robert G. Bonstein, Jr.
Vice President, First Consulting Group, Alpharetta, GA, USA
<rbonstein@fcgnet.com>

Joseph Casper
Vice President, First Consulting Group, Bellevue, WA, USA
<jcasper@fcgnet.com>

David Dimond
Technical Master, First Consulting Group, Boston, MA, USA
<ddimond@fcgnet.com>

Judith V. Douglas, MA, MHS
Associate, First Consulting Group, Baltimore, MD, USA
<jdouglas@fcgnet.com>

Michael Feyen
Senior Implementation Manager, First Consulting Group, Okemos, MI, USA
<mfeyen@fcgnet.com>

Michael Gorsage
Vice President and Managing Director, First Consulting Group, Alpharetta, GA, USA
<mgorsage@fcgnet.com>

Gordon Heinrich
Vice President, First Consulting Group, Oakland, CA, USA
<gheinrich@fcgnet.com>

Gail Hinte
Director, First Consulting Group, New York, NY, USA
<ghinte@fcgnet.com>

Barbara Hoehn
Vice President, First Consulting Group, New York, NY, USA
<bhoehn@fcgnet.com>

Tom Hurley
Vice President, First Consulting Group, Okemos, MI, USA
<thurley@fcgnet.com>

Richard N. Kramer
Vice President, First Consulting Group, Baltimore, MD, USA
<rkramer@fcgnet.com>

Philip Lohman, PhD
Director, First Consulting Group, Long Beach, CA, USA
<plohman@fcgnet.com>

Roice D. Luke, PhD
Professor and Director, Williamson Institute for Health Studies, Virginia Commonwealth University, Richmond, VA, USA
<luker@hsc.vcu.edu>

James R. McPhail
Director, First Consulting Group, Irving, TX, USA
<jmcphail@fcgnet.com>

Leslie Perreault
Director, First Consulting Group, New York, NY, USA
<lperreault@fcgnet.com>

Briggs T. Pille
Director, First Consulting Group, Chicago, IL, USA
<bpille@fcgnet.com>

James Reep
Chairman, First Consulting Group, Long Beach, CA, USA
<jreep@fcgnet.com>

Ramesh K. Shukla, PhD
Professor of Information Systems and Organizational Performance, Williamson Institute, Virginia Commonwealth University, Richmond, VA, USA
<shukla@hsc.vcu.edu>

Donald Tompkins
Vice President, First Consulting Group, Okemos, MI, USA
<dtompkins@fcgnet.com>

Tim Webb
Vice President, First Consulting Group, Alpharetta, GA, USA
<twebb@fcgnet.com>

Dale Will
Technical Master, First Consulting Group, Okemos, MI, USA
<dwill@fcgnet.com>

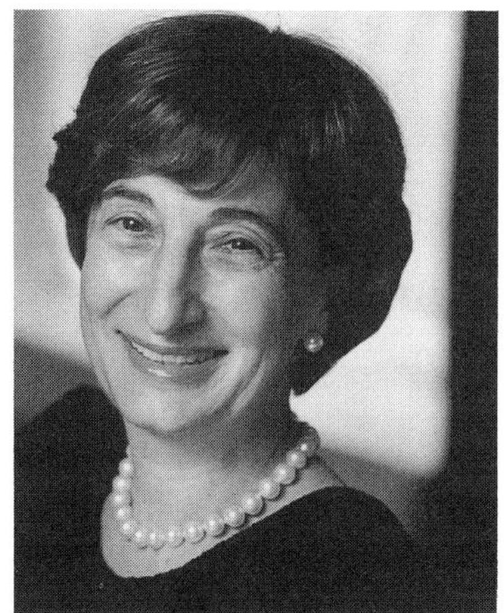

Marion J. Ball

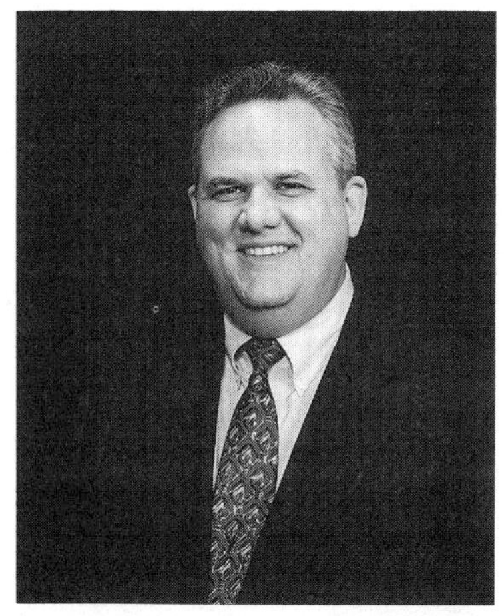

David Beaulieu

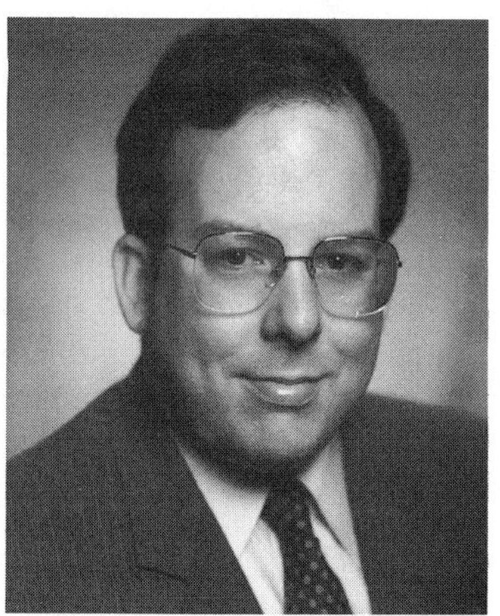

Robert G. Bonstein, Jr.

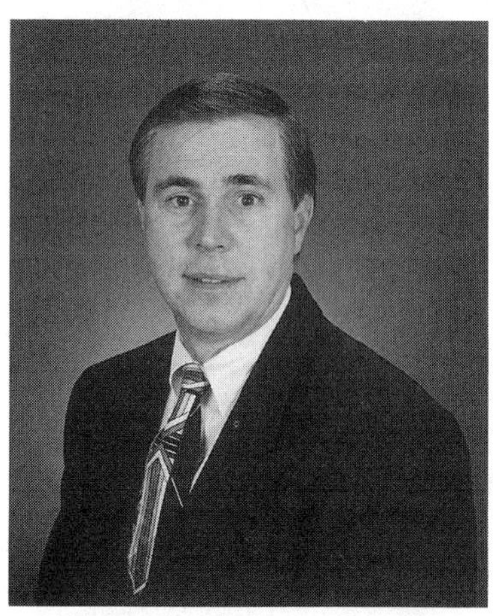

Joseph Casper

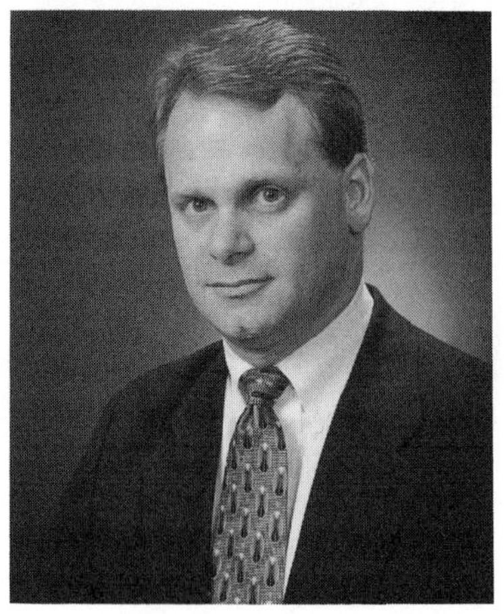

David Dimond

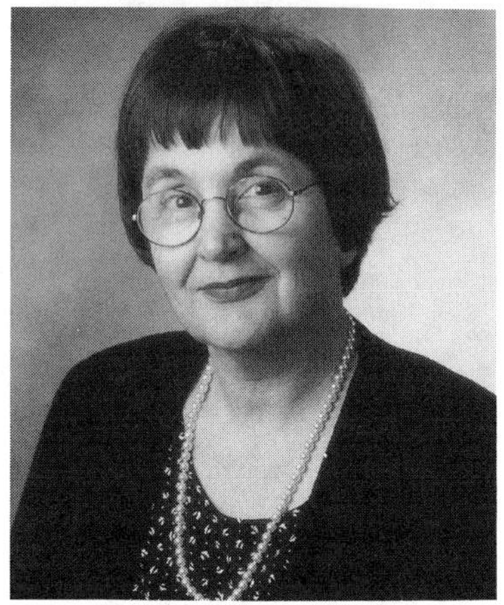

Judith V. Douglas

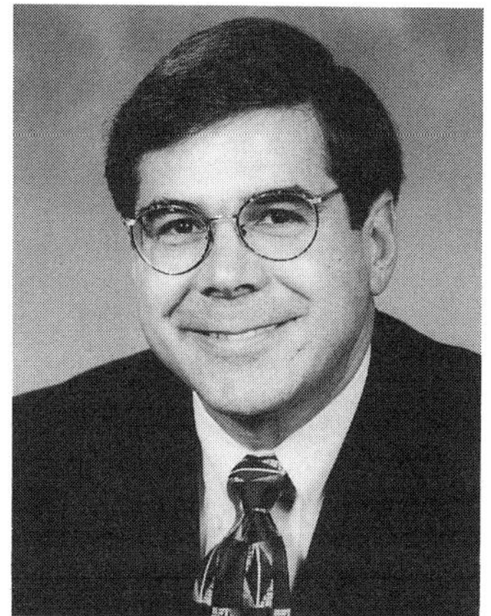
Michael Gorsage

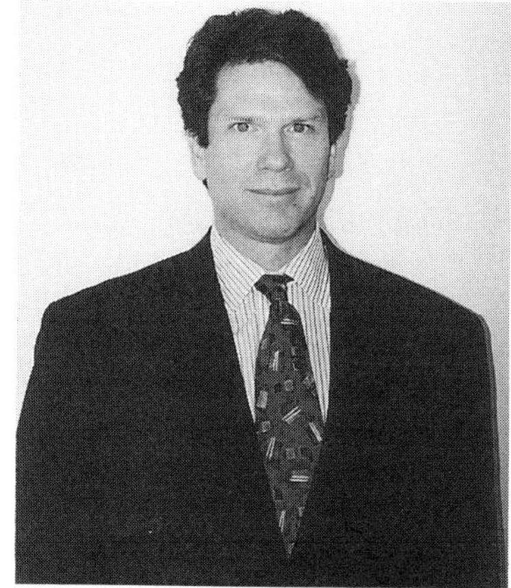
Gordon Heinrich

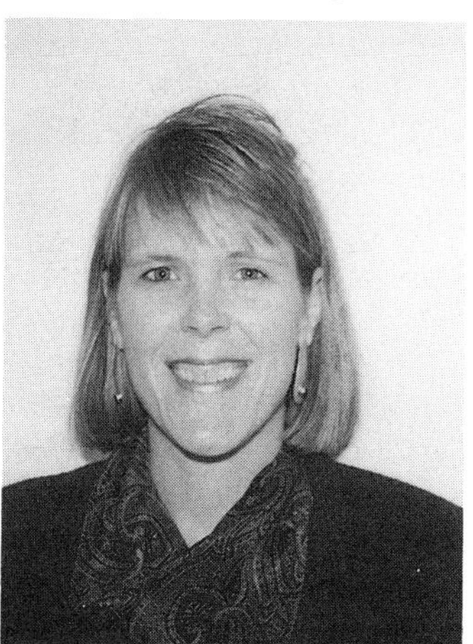
Gail Hinte

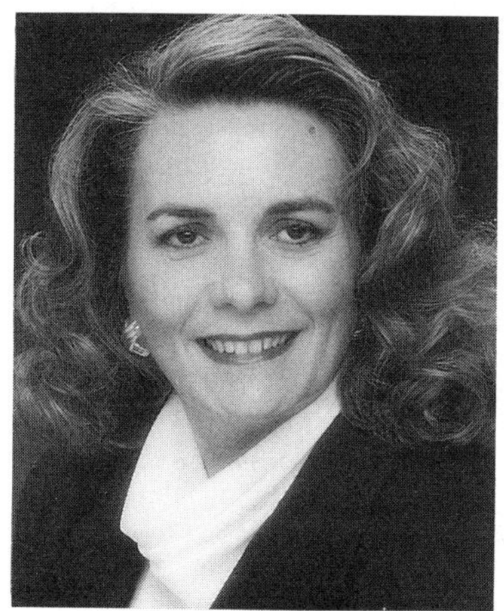
Barbara Hoehn

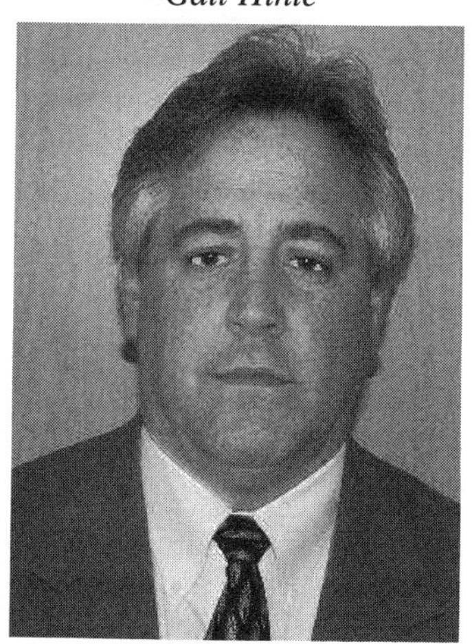
Tom Hurley

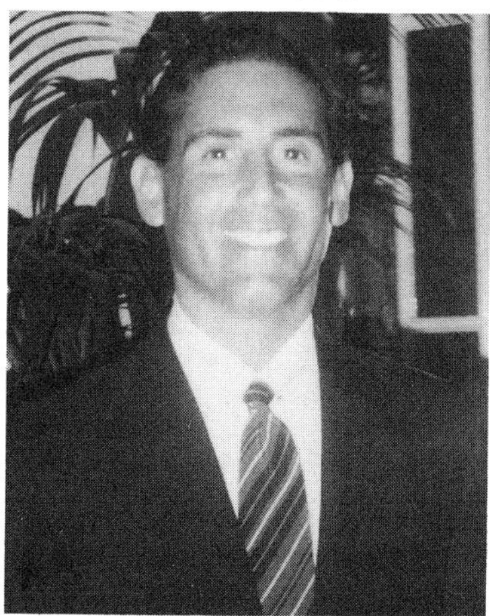
Richard N. Kramer

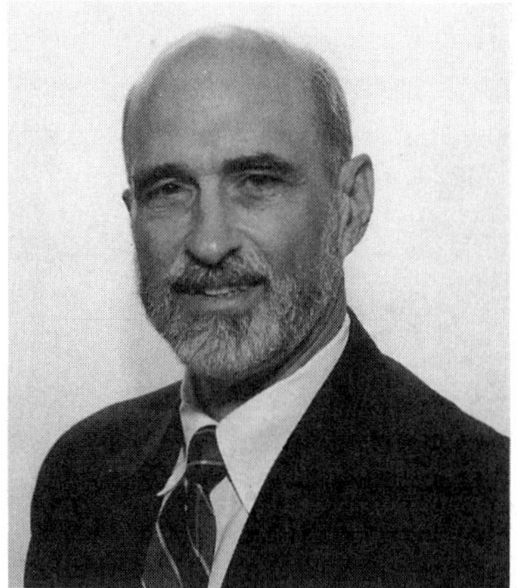

Philip Lohman

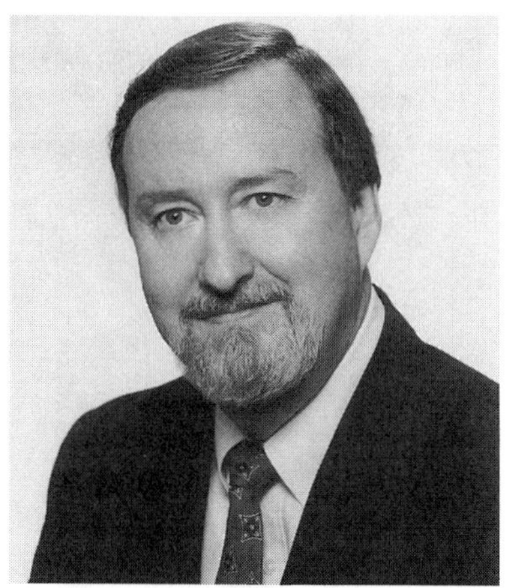

Roice D. Luke

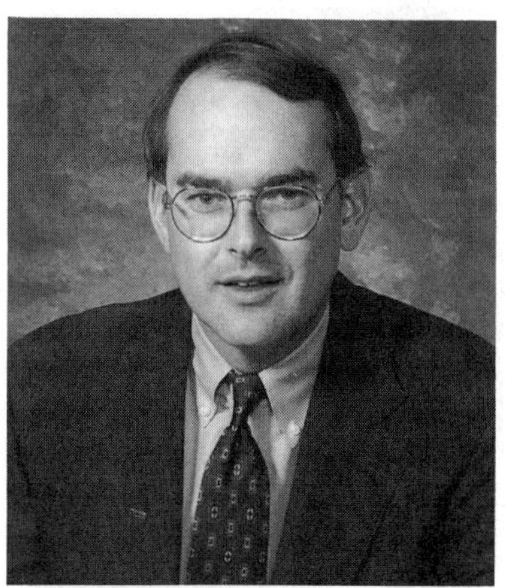

James R. McPhail

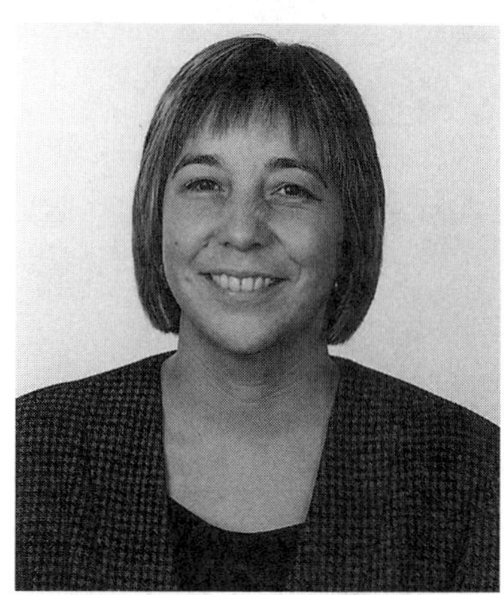

Leslie Perreault

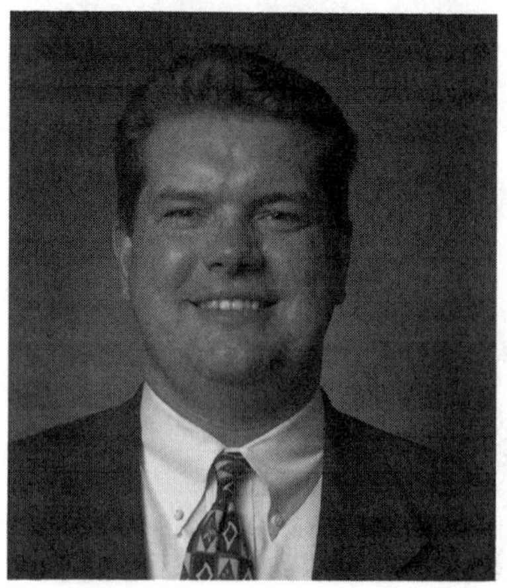

Briggs T. Pille

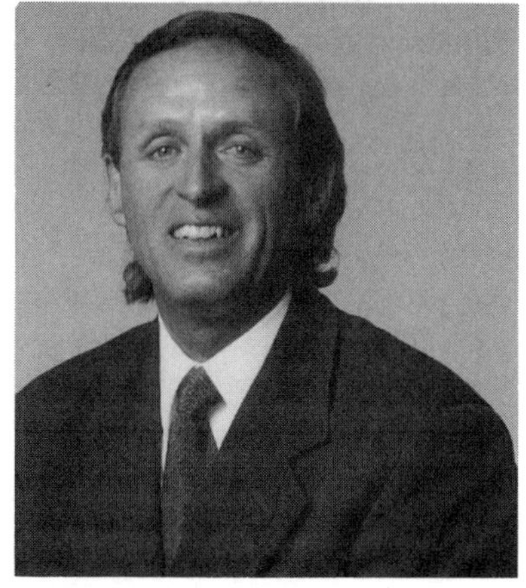

James Reep

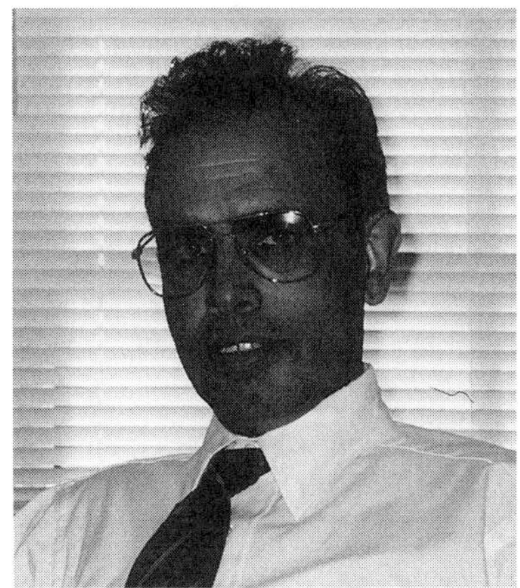

Ramesh K. Shukla

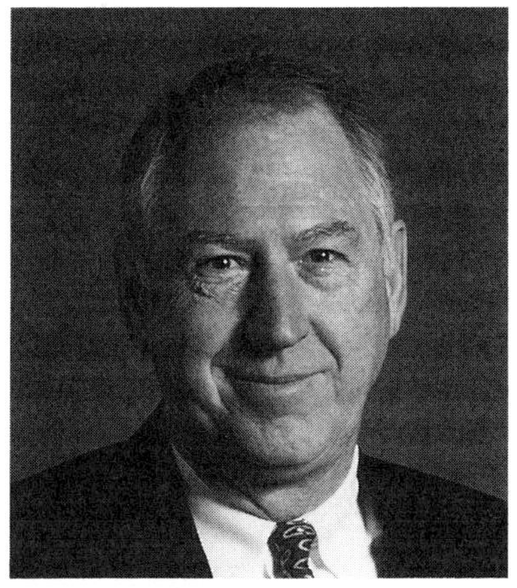

Donald Tompkins

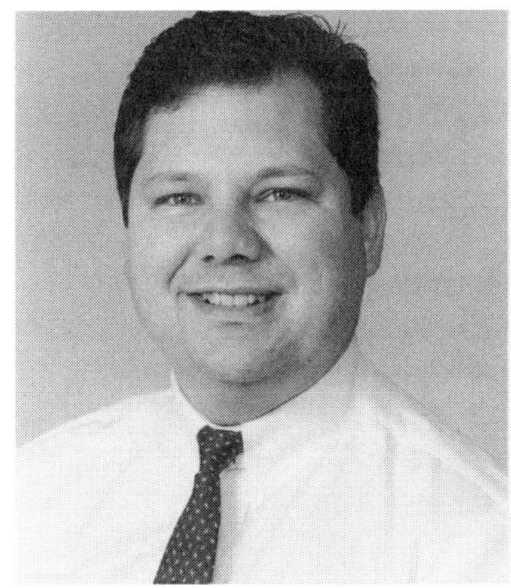

Tim Webb

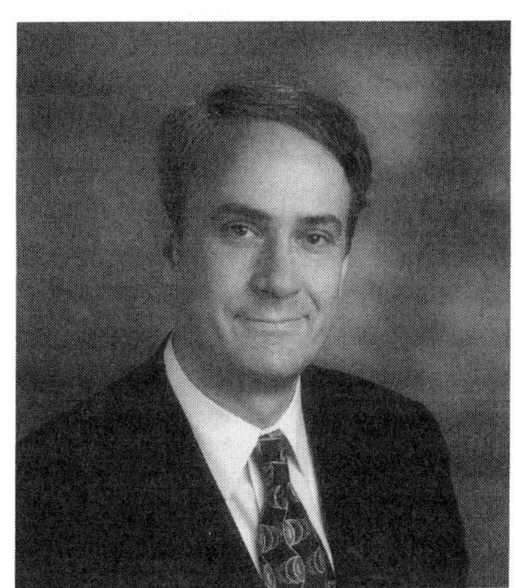

Dale Will

Health Informatics

(formerly Computers in Health Care)

Transforming Health Care Through Information
Case Studies
N.M. Lorenzi, R.T. Riley, M.J. Ball, and J.V. Douglas

Trauma Informatics
K.I. Maull and J.S. Augenstein

Filmless Radiology
E.L. Siegel and R.M. Kolodner

Knowledge Coupling
New Premises and New Tools for Medical Care and Education
L.L. Weed